Using Guided Imagery and Hypnosis in Brief Therapy and Palliative Care

Using Guided Imagery and Hypnosis in Brief Therapy and Palliative Care presents a model for effective single-session therapy.

Chapters include more than a dozen case studies with transcripts and commentary. Readers will learn how to use an adapted model of Remen's healing circle for preparing patients for surgery, and guided imagery and other approaches are presented for enhancing palliative care. Extensive appendixes provide a wide variety of valuable tools that psychotherapists can use with clients concerned with end-of-life issues.

Rubin Battino, LPCC, has published ten books on psychotherapy.

Using Guided Imagery and Hypnosis in Brief Therapy and Palliative Care

Rubin Battino

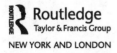

Routledge
Taylor & Francis Group

NEW YORK AND LONDON

First published 2021
by Routledge
52 Vanderbilt Avenue, New York, NY 10017

and by Routledge
2 Park Square, Milton Park, Abingdon, Oxon OX14 4RN

Routledge is an imprint of the Taylor & Francis Group, an informa business

Library of Congress Cataloging-in-Publication Data
A catalog record for this title has been requested

ISBN: 978-0-367-53848-4 (hbk)
ISBN: 978-0-367-53846-0 (pbk)
ISBN: 978-1-003-08805-9 (ebk)

Typeset in Times New Roman
by Newgen Publishing UK

Contents

Foreword

Michael Hoyt[1]

It is a pleasure to welcome this latest contribution, *Using Guided Imagery and Hypnosis in Brief Therapy and Palliative Care*, by Rubin Battino. As readers of his previous books (e.g., Battino, 2002, 2006, 2010, 2015; Battino & South, 2005) already know, he is wise and humane, clinically proficient, and skillful in explaining ways to use language to promote change effectively and efficiently. The terms *heal, whole, health, hale*, and *holy* all derive from the same old Middle English and Anglo-Saxon words (*hole, hale*). With great appreciation for our human capacity for hope and healing, Rubin shows us how to help our clients get there.

Most of what I've learned about the practice of psychotherapy has come from watching clinicians work (live or on video), from reading case studies and transcripts, and from observing and reflecting on my own clinical experiences. Sometimes the question is asked, "Is therapy art or science?" To my mind, the doing of therapy is a performance, an art and craft, a form of conversation probably closest to theater or drama. Some orienting theory can be useful and statistics may suggest some general trends, but the idiographic advantage of case studies is that the reader can learn what adept therapists, in fact, do in their clinical practices with real patients. As we all recognize, it is far different to read dry theoretical disquisitions than to see how talented clinicians actually function in their treatment interactions.

I have had the fortunate opportunity to watch Rubin work "live" as he has done guided imagery clinical demonstration interviews with clients at various conferences, and I am pleased that he has made available this book full of case material so that others can share these learning opportunities—including illustrations and thoughtful discussions of ways to use guided imagery and hypnosis in palliative care.

Underlying what he calls "chatting" is a passionate, highly skilled clinical awareness. This is a personal book—you get to meet the author as a person as well as an authority. He is a friend and a fine teacher. Readers will find their attention well rewarded.

Note

1 Michael F. Hoyt is a psychologist based in Mill Valley, CA. For more than three decades he was a staff member at the Kaiser Permanente Medical Center in San Rafael and Hayward, CA. He is a recipient of the APF Cummings Psyche Prize for lifetime contributions to the role of psychologists in organized healthcare. He has been honored as a Continuing Education Distinguished Speaker by both the American Psychological Association and the International Association of Marriage and Family Counselors, and as a Contributor of Note by the Milton H. Erickson Foundation. He has authored and edited numerous books (1995, 2000, 2004, 2009, 2014, 2017, 2019).

References

Battino, R. (2002). *Metaphoria: Metaphor and guided imagery for psychotherapy and healing*. Norwalk, CT: Crown House Publishing.

Battino, R. (2006). *Expectation: The very brief therapy book*. Bethel, CT: Crown House Publishing.

Battino, R. (2010). *Healing language: A guide for physicians, dentists, nurses, psychologists, social workers, and counselors*. Raleigh, NC: Lulu.com.

Battino, R. (2015). *When all else fails: Some new and some old tools for doing brief therapy*. Bethel, CT: Crown House Publishing.

Battino, R., & South, T.L. (2005). *Ericksonian approaches: A comprehensive manual* (2nd ed.). Bethel, CT: Crown House Publishing.

Foreword

Trevor Silvester[1]

I was having dinner with Rubin, early in our friendship, when he suddenly dropped into the conversation that he'd helped build a full scale accurate replica of the 1903 Wright Flyer.[2] This from a Professor of Chemistry, and one of the world's leading Ericksonian therapists. I had to ask, "Where on earth do you get the time for all this?" He looked up and dead-panned perfectly … "I don't dust." We should all be grateful for whoever does.

His being a chemist, perhaps it's not surprising that distillation is one of Rubin's great skills. "True refinement seeks simplicity." said Bruce Lee, and I've observed in all the masters I've observed or studied with, that as they age, they seem to do less while achieving more. So it is with Rubin, who is masterful in his use of Occam's razor, slicing away the inconsequentials of therapy to leave us with the hidden principles and, after such a distinguished and curious career, this book is packed with a refined wisdom that adds up to a monumental legacy.

In the modern therapy world, the expectation of many seems to be that success should be instant because they desire it to be so. They're easily lured into workshops and into courses that promise a quick and easy route to a lucrative living. Having taught would-be therapists for 20 years, I know they're doomed for deserved disappointment. Therapy rewards service to humanity, and that comes from learning your trade. It takes effort, a tolerance for disappointment and frustration, and the consistency and persistence to become great at something. Somewhere in the process you let go of ego, and when you have, success will more easily find you. Chase it with your ego and it all too often runs away. I mention this because the thing that made an impression on me when I experienced Rubin's teaching was his humility. He stood in front of us, opened his brain, and just quietly shared it with us without fuss or fanfare, and it's been so every time I've had the pleasure of learning from him. Perhaps working with the chronic and terminally ill does that through burning away the ego and leaving what's really important about being a therapist—the sacred privilege of helping someone find their way ahead.

So, in this book you'll find an absence of ego, but a ton of things to learn, simply shared. Well, as simply shared as a Professor of Chemistry will allow—the footnotes alone deserve another book. What struck me the most as I made my way through the pages was the breadth of Rubin's knowledge and experience. This really isn't a book it's possible to rush through, there is simply too much good information and advice to absorb. In the chapter on hypnotic language several of Kay Thompson's quotes made me have to go and lie down! And whatever your level of experience, the many case studies are an opportunity to learn from his lean language, his pacing, his deep simplicity.

This is a book compiled by an aging magpie, who has flown far and wide, driven by his curiosity and desire to find what is shiny in therapy. We are lucky to have a magpie who has sorted the gold from the brass, and arranged what is left into the most pleasing arrangement for those of us who are similarly curious. This is knowledge shared for the simple good of sharing. This is a book for the eternal student, striving to be better today than yesterday. This is a book to remind us of what it takes to be great at what we do. It's been my honor to write about it, as it's been my pleasure and privilege to be his friend.

Notes

1   Trevor Silvester is a practicing hypnotherapist in England. He was for some years the editor of the UK *Hypnotherapy Journal*. He is a Fellow of the UK National Council for Hypnotherapy and the Hypnotherapy Society. Silvester is the founder and training director of The Quest Institute, a company that runs courses in Cognitive Therapy (Silvester, 2010) and Neuro Linguistic Programming. His two books on "wordweaving" (2003, 2006) are fascinating and enlightening and practical. (His books are available from Amazon.com.)

2   RB note: this is now hanging in the atrium of the Wright State University library in Dayton, OH.

Preface

In a way this book is the culmination of my life's work as a volunteer and facilitator and therapist with people who have life-challenging diseases, and also for caregivers. Much of what is in this book can be used by practicing psychotherapists with their regular client population, especially the adaptation of the guided imagery model to psychotherapy. I am a follower of the work of Milton H. Erickson, MD, and so much of what is written here is connected with hypnosis and the various forms of psychotherapy he pioneered. Chapter 26 on guided imagery and hypnosis and other approaches for palliative care distills much of my life's work.

Over 30 years ago I read Bernie Siegel's first book, *Love, Medicine & Miracles* (1986). After finishing reading this inspiring and eye-opening book I asked myself why I as a therapist with a fair number of people skills, was not using those skills to help people who had life-challenging diseases. So, I tracked down an ECaP (Exceptional Cancer Patients) group in the Dayton area (not far from where I live). I was invited to attend their semi-monthly meetings, which were held at Hospice of Dayton. (They were not affiliated with Hospice of Dayton who kindly provided them with a meeting room. There will be more about this group and how it works in Chapter 2.) My involvement with the members of this group and with individuals I worked with taught me a great deal about end-of-life issues, how they affected people, and what would be useful in spending time with them. A diagnosis of a life-challenging disease inevitably leads people to think about what is *really important* to them. This was always something we explored together or in groups. This exploration almost always came up with the following two discoveries: the first was that people and relationships were primary; and the second was an involvement with Nature. *Life is with people.* Life also involves how we relate to the world around us, the earth, the sky, the heavens, the forests, the plains, and all of the myriad bodies of water.

An inevitable part of my volunteer work is that many of the people I got to know deeply and well died. There was sadness, feelings of emptiness and loss, and also the realization that I got to spend time with many remarkable people. They each enriched my life in different ways. There was courage and despair, hope and depression, hopelessness and imagination, dreams and discoveries. I look back and marvel at how amazing each of them was in their own way—we are all unique and each of us is a miracle. I was honored by their willingness to spend time with me, and by their openness and sharing. I am writing this now (2017) at a time when I learned yesterday that someone I knew well, and with whom I was able to share many experiences, died suddenly of an accident at age 68. So, tomorrow morning I will attend her funeral service. When this happens there is always the regret of why did I not call her and arrange to have lunch with her so we could just chat? I (and we) put off those calls and contacts when we believe that the other person will always be around. At this time, too, my oldest friend, George (from high school days), is dying of cancer 2000 miles away in California. I call and chat regularly with him and his wife. Sometimes, that has to be enough ... [Note: I started writing this book over three years ago in 2017, and George died soon after I wrote the preceding. It is now three years later, five of my friends in Yellow Springs where I live have also died. And, as of this writing (November 2019) my brother Ralph, who was my remaining sibling, died in his hundredth year in March. This is what accompanies us as we age.]

The books I have written that are related to psychotherapy contained few case studies, although there were appropriate illustrative scripts in many of them. I recently had Case Study 1 published, and I decided that I would include in this book 16 case studies. They are interspersed between some of the chapters. I also chose to use many of these case studies as vehicles to discuss relevant therapeutic approaches. Since I spent 38 years of my life as a full-time academic, and I love doing training in psychotherapy-related areas, I could not resist making this book a text in large part. When I gave chemistry lectures and did psychotherapy workshops and teaching and training it was my practice to more than less follow the syllabus or the Power Point. On the other hand, whenever what I was talking about led to other ideas or thoughts or stories, I would just digress to talk about them. I found over the years that my students and many of the listeners at workshops, etc., remembered the stories and digressions more than the "straight" material. So, I have given myself permission to do the same thing here (although sometimes I sneak these digressions into footnotes!). All of the epigraphs opening each chapter (except one) are my own three-line poems, and were selected to go with the contents of that chapter.

Although in the beginning of this Preface I indicated that much of the book would be about my volunteer work, I decided that the chapter I originally wrote on end-of-life issues would better fit in as an appendix (B) so I have moved it there. As an introduction to that appendix (A) I have included an essay I wrote recently entitled "Ruminations on Turning 88." My hope in doing this is that the reader will discover many comments that will lead him/her to ruminations of their own in terms of what is important in their lives and also about unthought of imperatives controlling their life choices and activities. The other appendices have been included either because they are connected to earlier material in this book, or just because I like them in terms of having special meaning in my life.

I have a number of special friends, and I want them to know that I deeply appreciate their friendship and support over the years: Carl Hammerschlag, MD, John D. Lentz, D. Min., Rob McNeilly, MD, Eric Greenleaf, PhD, Roxanna Erickson Klein, PhD, Ernest L. Rossi. PhD, Carlos Casanova, MS, and Trevor Silvester and his wife, Bex. I am also indebted to all of the people I have met in my volunteer work as they have taught me much about both living, end-of-life issues and dying. My psychotherapy clients have been a great source of practical knowledge.

In writing this book I have had the support of Charlotte (my wife of 60+ years) whom I deeply love and appreciate, and also that of our two sons, their wives, and our eight grandchildren. I owe a special thanks to Michael F. Hoyt, PhD, who has read the manuscript in its many stages, and provided guidance along with innumerable helpful suggestions. He is an exceptional person, friend, and colleague. I also thank Dan Short, PhD, for many helpful suggestions.

Rubin Battino
Yellow Springs, OH
April 2020

1   Introduction

Expectation, the Placebo Effect, and Chatting

> ground fog luminous
> and the moon in the morning
> a single bird sings

1.1 Expectation

A number of years ago I heard Steve de Shazer talk about a research project
they carried out at the Brief Family Therapy Center of Milwaukee. They did
a lot of research, and their clients were anyone who walked into their office.
Being located in the inner city meant their clients were diverse and frequently
difficult to work with. The particular research I cite here had to do with the
expectation of the client. There was an intake form to be filled out. The receptionist, when looking over the form, said to the client something like, "Oh,
from what you have written here it usually takes our staff about five sessions
to help people." The next client would be told ten sessions. The staff were not
told about this, that is, they did not know which client was told five and which
ten, and they did not know that this was going on. (After all, the receptionist
really had no idea of how many sessions a particular client would need based
on what they had written!) About one year later the staff were informed about
this project and were asked to look at their notes for their clients. They were
specifically asked about how many sessions they had with each client, and
when the client started doing "significant" work. The results were fascinating
in that the clients who were told five sessions typically started doing significant change work around the fourth session, and the ones told ten sessions
around the eighth or ninth session. Note that the therapists did not all work
the same way, i.e., from the same theoretical or practical orientations. The
conclusion that the researchers (and I) drew from this experiment is that the
expectation of the client plays a major role in how effective therapy is, and
how many sessions are needed.

As a scientist it seemed to me that if I graphed these results and the clients
were told one session that this would make a significant impact on how fast
you could do effective therapy. So, I tell all of my clients that *my expectation*

is that we will be able to do significant change work in the first session, and that I work as if every session were the last one. I also tell them that the decision to return is theirs, and I will always schedule another appointment at their request. I rarely see clients more than one time. Since I work for myself my sessions are always open-ended: the average length of a session is about 90 minutes.

There is a great deal of literature on single-session therapy (SST) and very brief therapy. The first book in this area was the one by Talmon (1990); the subtitle was *Maximizing the Effect of the First (and Often Only) Therapeutic Encounter*. Talmon worked at Kaiser Permanente in the San Francisco Bay Area and studied with Michael Hoyt and Robert Rosenbaum the work of some 30 psychiatrists, psychologists, and social workers for a 12-month period. Here are the significant results:

- To the best of my knowledge, the "founder" of single-session therapy (SST) was none other than Sigmund Freud, better known as the founder of the longest form of psychotherapy, psychoanalysis. At the end of the nineteenth century, Freud treated a patient known as Katharina in a single session during one of his vacations on an Austrian mountaintop. Later, he reported to have cured the composer Gustav Mahler's impotence during a single long walk in the woods. (p. 3)
- When I studied the data, I was astonished by what I found: (1) the modal (most frequent) length of therapy for every one of the therapists was a single session, and (2) 30 per cent of all patients chose to come for only one session in a period of one year. (p. 7)
- … the therapeutic orientation of the therapists had no impact on the percentage of SSTs in their total practice. (p. 7)
- I later studied 100,000 scheduled outpatient appointments during a five-year period (1983–1088) and found the frequency of SSTs to be extremely consistent. (p. 7)
- Of all of the SST patients contacted, 88 per cent reported either "much improvement" or "improvement" since the session (on a five-point scale); … and 65 per cent reported either having positive changes that were clearly unrelated to the presenting problem and might be attributed to a ripple effect. The SST patients showed slightly more improvement and more satisfaction than the patients who were seen for more therapy, but the differences were not significant. (p. 16)

The subsequent book edited by Hoyt and Talmon (2014) entitled *Capturing the Moment. Single Session Therapy and Walk-in Services* contains some 25 chapters by authors working in these fields. This is a treasure of information on the current status of the SST field. Interestingly, there are descriptions of walk-in single session facilities in Canada, the United States, Mexico,

Australia, China, Sweden, Haiti, Italy, and Cambodia. Another recent book, *Single-Session Therapy by Walk-in or Appointment* (edited by Hoyt, Bobele, Slive, Young, & Talmon, 2018) provides even more evidence that brief and single-session therapies work. A related and useful book is the one by Hoyt (2009) entitled *Brief Psychotherapies. Principles & Practices*. The more recent book by Hoyt (2017) is entitled *Brief Therapy and Beyond. Stories, Language, Love, Hope, and Time*.[1]

In the next section I write about how the essence of SST—expectation—is based on the placebo effect.

1.2 The Placebo Effect

The essence of how the placebo effect works is via the *expectation* of the listener or receiver that whatever is being said or being done will be effective. In fact, the history of healing and curing (distinctions made later) is the history of the placebo effect. In prehistoric times (and continuing to the present in various cultures) mental or physical illness was believed to be caused by the mind or the body being "possessed" by evil spirits. Thus, you can find skulls with holes drilled in them from prehistoric times. The belief then was that by drilling a hole in the skull (trephining) that the evil spirit would be let out. For physical ailments, the causing agent (or spirit) would be removed from the body by: bloodletting, purgatives, sudorifics (cause or increase sweating), emetics and enemas, or cupping (attaching heated glass cups to the back— these cups can still be purchased online!). In the recent movie *Victoria and Abdul* Queen Victoria's physician frequently asks for stool samples so he can study them. Not too long ago there were advocates of "colonic cleansing" to cure cancers. On the other hand, the modern medical practice of doing urine and blood analyses and tests of fecal samples are backed up with scientific studies that show that these tests can and do provide useful medical information. There are many cultures and religions who practiced various versions of *exorcism* for both mental and physical ailments. All of these methods depend on the belief and expectation of both the practitioners and the patients that these "cleansings" are effective.

There is a vast literature on the placebo effect, and I am only going to cite one source here (and a few more in the section on the nocebo effect): Shapiro and Shapiro (1997). (Chapter 4 in my book on guided imagery [Battino (2000)] is on the placebo effect.) The word " placebo," Latin for "I will please." dates back to a Latin translation of the Bible by St Jerome. Shapiro and Shapiro's preferred definition (p. 41) is:

> A placebo is any therapy (or that component of any therapy) that is intentionally or knowingly used for the nonspecific, psychological, or psychophysiological, therapeutic effect, or that is used for a presumed therapeutic

effect on a patient, symptom, or illness but is without specific activity for the condition being treated.

The Shapiros have categorically stated that until recently the history of Western medicine (physical and mental) has been the history of the placebo effect. That is, it was not until the 1950s that there were double-blind studies for physical effects. It has long been known, of course, that opium was useful for controlling pain. However, the purity and dosage of this substance was not studied clinically until the 1950s and later. There was also a great deal of folk medicine that was used, and that appeared to help people. In the history of the development of folk cures many people got ill or died from experimenting! It appears that humans are predisposed to the belief that healers will be helpful (this belief, of course, is useful to all healers, medical and psychological and religious).

There are various factors that enhance the placebo effect in medicine. It has been shown, for example, that if you take the "standard" size of a pill to be that of an aspirin, that both smaller *and* larger placebo pills have been found to be more effective simply due to their size. In addition, placebo injections are more effective than pills. Pharmaceutical companies have sold (and still sell) placebos for medical purposes in many sizes, colors, and shapes. When a new drug or procedure is introduced, the publicity (and enthusiasm of the purveyors) leads to that treatment to be more effective initially, and decreases as time moves on. The U.S. is only one of two "advanced" countries (the other is New Zealand) that permits the advertising of prescription medicines on TV. The TV ads have to include warnings about side effects—if you listen to the horrors that can possibly ensue from taking that new medicine, no one in their right mind would take it or ask their doctor to prescribe it! Sadly, these ads appear to be effective in promoting those meds, possibly because viewers pay more attention to the lively and active actors who have presumably taken that medicine!

It has only been in recent times that psychotherapeutic methods have been studied carefully enough to have some of them shown to be clinically effective. Wikipedia, for example, states the following about cognitive behavioral therapy:

> Cognitive behavioral therapy (CBT) is a psychosocial intervention that is the most widely used *evidence-based practice* for improving mental health. Guided by empirical research, CBT focuses on the development of personal coping strategies that target solving current problems and changing unhelpful patterns in cognitions (e.g. thoughts, beliefs, and attitudes), behaviors, and emotional regulation. It was originally designed to treat depression, and is now used for a number of mental health conditions.

(Italics added)

The practitioners of "evidence-based" methods have an advantage in working with clients in that they can cite this, thus *implying* an expectation that this method is more effective than other methods. In addition, insurance coverage appears to favor evidence-based approaches. Perhaps, the bottom line here is that the therapist's expectation (however communicated to a client) helps outcomes.

1.3 Other and Related Expectational Phenomena

Hahn (1997) has written about the *nocebo effect* where expectation is used to harm people. Two quotes follow:

- The nocebo effect is the causation of sickness (or death) by expectation of sickness (or death) and by associated emotional states. There are two forms of the nocebo effect. In the *specific* form, the subject experiences a particular negative outcome and that outcome subsequently occurs. ... In the *generic* form, subjects have vague negative expectations. (p. 56)
- The nocebo phenomenon is a little-recognized facet of culture that may be responsible for a substantial variety of pathology around the world. However, the extent of the phenomenon is not yet known, and evidence is piecemeal and ambiguous. (p. 71)

Commonly known examples of the nocebo effect are in " voodoo" deaths, and the Australian Aborigine practice of "pointing the bone." In addition, many cultures contain nocebos in terms of the "evil eye" and possession by " evil spirits."

A particularly difficult nocebo effect is the one resulting from a medical doctor (or other medical personnel) inadvertently making statements (sometimes called " hex" or " witch" messages) such as:

- You've got breast cancer, and it's going to kill you. [Note: this is an actual message a friend of mine got over the phone from her doctor!]
- There is nothing more we can do for you medically.
- At this stage, it can only get worse.
- Look, you're just going to have to live with it.
- Listen, just enjoy what's left of the rest of your life.
- I'm so sorry!

As another example, Thomas (1987) reported that patients did appreciably less well than a control group if a physician told them, "I am not sure what is the matter with you, and I am not sure the treatment will have an effect." Please note that these statements are by and large medically accurate prognoses. Yet, the effect is that of a nocebo message, which closes down hope and possibilities. Again, there is an overt or hidden noxious message in them.[2]

To provide further background on both the placebo and nocebo effects I am simply going to cite here a number of recent papers on these subjects by their authors and titles (the full reference to each paper is in the reference section at the end of this book).

1 Colloca and Benedetti (2005). "Placebos as pain killers: is mind as real as matter?"
2 Colloca and Benedetti (2006). "How prior experience shapes placebo analgesia."
3 Benedetti, Lanotte, Lopiano, and Colloca (2007). (Review) "When words are painful: unraveling the mechanisms of the placebo effect."
4 Colloca and Benedetti (2007). "Nocebo analgesia: how anxiety is turned into pain."
5 Enck, Benedetti, and Schedlowski (2008). "New insights into the placebo and nocebo responses."
6 Miller and Colloca (2009). "The legitimacy of placebo treatments in clinical practice: evidence and ethics."
7 Finniss, Kaptchuk, Miller, and Benedetti (2010). "Biological, clinical, and ethical advances of placebo effects."
8 Tinnermann, Geuter, Sprenger, Finsterbusch, and Buchel (2017). "Interactions between the brain and spinal cord mediate value effects in nocebo hyperalgesia."
9 Colloca (2017). "Nocebo effects can make you feel the pain."

A related phenomenon, *nosocomial infections*, is described by Wikipedia as:

> A hospital-acquired infection (HAI), also known as a nosocomial infection, is an infection that is acquired in a hospital or other health care facility. To emphasize both hospital and nonhospital settings, it is sometimes instead called a health care-associated infection (HAI or HCAI). ... Such an infection can be acquired in hospital, nursing home, rehabilitation facility, outpatient clinic, or other clinical settings. In the United States, the Centers for Disease Control and Prevention estimated roughly 1.7 million hospital-associated infections, from all types of microorganisms, including bacteria and fungi combined, cause or contribute to 99,000 deaths each year.

Nosocomial also applies to medical facility caused mistakes and diseases in addition to infections. This is an incredible number, and these infections can be prevented by appropriate hygienic practices. When I required a knee replacement several years ago I checked the infection rate at all of my local hospitals (this information is available) and found to my astonishment that all of them had infection rates of about 10–13%. Of course, there are hospitals that pay strict attention to hygiene, the most common form is having all people who interact with patients actively scrub and wash their hands before contacting the patient in any way. Where proper hygiene is practiced the infection rates are typically below 1%.

Again, here is Wikipedia information on iatrogenic and iatrogenesis (both are considered to be nosocomial):

> Iatrogenesis (from the Greek for "brought forth by the healer") refers to any effect on a person, resulting from any activity of one or more persons acting as healthcare professionals or promoting products or services as beneficial to health, that does not support a goal of the person affected. Globally as of 2013 an estimated 20 million negative effects from treatment occurred. It is estimated that 142,000 people died in 2013 from adverse effects of medical treatment up from 94,000 in 1990. The term iatrogenic is defined as "induced in a patient by a physician's activity, manner, or therapy. Used especially to pertain to a complication of treatment." Furthermore, these estimates of death due to error are lower than those in a recent Institutes of Medicine report. If the higher estimates are used, the deaths due to iatrogenic causes would range from 230,000 to 284,000. Even at the lower estimate of 225,000 deaths per year, this constitutes the third leading cause of death in the U.S.

This is another incredible bit of information. On the other hand, patients on intake are given a wrist bracelet that has their name and birthday on it to prevent mis-identification. It is also protective to have an advocate with you who can take notes and look out for your welfare.

With respect to expectation, nosocomial and iatrogenetic phenomena are *not* nocebo connected—you just need to know about their existence.

1.4 Comments on Disease/Cure and Illness/Heal

I find it helpful to make a distinction between disease and illness even though generally they are thought to be the same. To me, a *disease* is something that is physically wrong in the body. That is, it is not normal health to have an ulcer, cancer, a broken bone, or an infection. Modern medicine is quite good in returning the body to normalcy via medicines and treatments like antibiotics and setting bones. My right knee was in awful shape and I had a full knee replacement about 11 years ago. So, I was "cured" of that disease. Thus, to me, diseases are *cured*. Whatever is physically wrong has been corrected and the body returned to normalcy.

I define an *illness* as what we *feel* and *think* and *believe* about the disease. What do we think about it? What does it mean to us? What we feel about the disease is generally determined by our upbringing, the culture in which we grow up, and in many instances by our religious beliefs. So, I pair *illness* with *healing*. Changing how we feel about the disease also changes our attitudes and actions, and frequently results in feeling calmer and better about our-selves, and more able to cope and live with the disease. When someone gets a diagnosis of cancer it is not unusual to get depressed and feel both hopeless and helpless. These emotions can have deleterious effects on our health and our ability to enhance curing treatments. In my experience working as a volunteer with people who have life-challenging diseases, I have found that healing (changing how one feels about the disease) can have positive physical effects and aid in cures.

It is also important to distinguish the magnitude of pain from how we react to it. Thus, it is useful to have two scales. The first one is, "On a scale of zero to ten where zero is complete comfort with no pain and ten is the most excruciating pain you have had or can think about, what are you feeling now?" The second one is, "On a scale of zero to ten, how much is this *bothering* you now?" You may have a pain of 7.3, and it only bothers you at a 3.1 level. Or, you might have a pain of 2.7 that bothers you at an 8.4 level. That is, for example, hangnails may have a low pain level but can be very bothersome. Also, it is not unusual for a person to experience a strong pain level, but one to which they have become somewhat inured. A surgeon I know told me that he uses these two scales all of the time (after he read about them in my book on healing language (Battino, 2010)) and finds this quite useful.

Psychotherapy, counseling, and groups have all been effective in this healing work. In the next chapter I shall discuss the way that the Charlie Brown Group of Exceptional Patients and Caregivers works.

1.5 RB's Model of Therapy, the Therapeutic Alliance, and Chatting

A. RB's Model of Therapy

I have a simple model of how therapy works. Clients come to see us for help because they are stuck. That is, there is some stimulus in their lives that typ-ically results in one response, behavior, or interpretation. They are stuck in being depressed, overweight, compulsive, anxious, etc. Our job then is to guide them into discovering other ways of responding, behaving, and/or interpreting. That is, to provide them with the opportunity of choosing other ways of living. We do this by telling stories, guiding them through something like the Miracle Question, having them do ambiguous function assignments or therapeutic ordeals, and reframing as a few examples. The bottom line is to get them to *do something different* in terms of their thinking and/or actions. It is to have them realize and experience *choice* in their lives.

One of the simplest "shock" treatments involving choice is an *inclusivity* statement like, "I wonder what it would be like to be happily depressed or sloppily organized or aggressively cautious or calmly excited?" These paired emotions are oxymoronic and open up ways of thinking and behaving that are new, and a bit startling and confusing. Perhaps the most useful method of suggesting choice is reframing in which you help the client perceive actions and feelings from other perspectives.

In subsequent chapters many choice interventions will be illustrated and discussed in detail. Again, our job is being conveyors of choice.

B. The Therapeutic Alliance

Before discussing the importance of therapeutic alliance it is useful to think about the interaction of two people who meet for the first time. There are, of course, expectations on both the part of the client and the therapist. The client expects assistance in getting out of his/her stuck place, and the therapist expects his/her skills and knowledge to facilitate such a change (or changes). A typical session is 50 to 60 minutes (mine are usually 90 minutes or more). So, out of that day of 24 hours when the client is awake for 16 hours you are with him/her for about 6% of their day, or less than 1% of their week. If your clients are in their 30s, 40s, or 50s, then you are spending with them a minuscule part of their lives. Even if you do an extensive history on intake, you will only be informed of a few specific highlights. Assuming your opening questions are focused on *why* they have come to see you, then you only get a brief glimpse of all of the history leading up to that moment. Thus, given how little we can actually know about the person seated in front of us, we somehow have to find ways of connecting with them, building trust and confidence, and *guiding* them to satisfactory outcomes. This is a truly monumental endeavor! So, how is it possible that the literature shows that therapy works (really helps people)? The answers may be that the session is focused on immediate and narrow concerns, and that well-trained therapists are able to obtain their client's trust and confidence in a very short time. This comes under rapport building skills and the therapeutic alliance.

Here are some relevant comments by Tyler and Wampold (2012) on the "real relationship," expectation, and connections:

> there are characteristics of the therapist that foster trust. For example, racial/ethnic minorities[3] prefer therapists of the same racial or ethnic group and rate those therapists more positively. The concept of the "expertness" of the therapist has been a factor in the initial formation of the alliance. ... research has shown that individuals have an expectation that a therapist must display a level of expertness in order to facilitate change. ... Empathy has been found to be a consistent predictor of therapy outcome.
>
> (p. 606)

What is missing in the discussion of the real relationship is how it works to produce benefits—how is it therapeutic? We assert that the main way positive outcomes are achieved through the real relationship is through the salutary effects of being *connected* to another human being, particularly one who is invested in the other's well-being.

(p. 608, italics added)

The importance of expectations for humans is in some ways self-evident. The human brain is designed for the past and future as well as the present. That is, humans can recall the past in vivid imagery, as well as anticipate the future. The expectations created thereby have powerful effects not only in the mind but on the body. The power of expectations becomes evident from examining the effects of placebos on humans.

(p. 614)

A definition of the therapeutic relationship (also called the therapeutic alliance, the helping alliance, or the working alliance) refers to the relationship between a healthcare professional and a client. It is the means by which a therapist and a client hope to engage with each other, and effect beneficial change in the client. There is a vast literature on this subject, which I recently dipped into before writing this section. In fact, there is research to show that a determination of trustworthiness is made within seconds of seeing a face! I only cite from a few more papers.

The first is an article by Norcross and Wampold (2011) summarizing the work in a special issue of *Psychotherapy*. The title of the Norcross and Wampold article is, "Evidence-Based Therapy Relationships: Research Conclusions and Clinical Practices." The abstract states in part (p. 98):

In this closing article of this special issue, we present the conclusions and recommendations of the interdivisional task force on evidence-based therapy relationships. The work was based on series of meta-analyses conducted on the effectiveness of various relationship elements and methods of adaptation. A panel of experts concluded that several relationship elements were demonstrably effective (alliance in individual psychotherapy, alliance in youth psychotherapy, alliance in family therapy, …).

The second article is by Wampold (2015) and is entitled, "How Important Are the Common Factors in Psychotherapy. An Update." The abstract states:

The common factors have a long history in the field of psychotherapy theory, research and practice. To understand the evidence supporting them as important therapeutic elements, the contextual model of psychotherapy is outlined. Then the evidence, primarily from meta-analyses, is presented for particular common factors, including alliance, empathy, expectations, cultural adaptation, and therapist differences. Then the evidence for four factors related to specificity, including treatment differences, specific ingredients, adherence, and competence is presented. The evidence supports the conclusion that the common factors are important for producing the benefits of psychotherapy.

From my perspective it is significant that alliance and expectation are effective. The literature varies widely on how effective they are. I have seen results where the effectiveness of the therapeutic alliance accounts for 7% to much higher values (like above 50%). In my private practice clients know that *my* expectation is that we will need only one session to help them get what they want out of therapy. (They know that I will always see them at their request for additional sessions.) How I currently implement the therapeutic alliance is discussed in the next section.

C. Chatting

As an introduction to chatting (see Chapter 21 for a longer exposition), which is my preferred way of functioning now, the following quote from Tyler and Wampold (2012) on empathy is useful (p. 610):

> We argue that empathy is another evolved mechanism that enables psychotherapy to be in the context of the real relationship. Empathy is a complex process by which an individual can be affected by and share the emotional state of another, assess the reasons for another's state, and identify with the other being by adopting his or her perspective. Empathy has many purposes. It allows beings to rapidly and automatically understand the emotional states of other beings and is in turn necessary for the regulation of cooperation, goal sharing, and social interactions.

I have been trained in and studied many approaches to doing psychotherapy. Currently the main thing I do is very brief therapy, and usually incorporate into it a hypnosis session. My orientation in using hypnosis is mainly derived from the work of Milton H. Erickson, MD. Over the years I have evolved into doing something I call "chatting." My intake form is short and simple and ends with space for the client to give a "brief statement of concern(s), and what you want out of counseling." (Please note that I am a licensed professional clinical counselor in the State of Ohio.) My clients know that I consider each session to be the last one, and that they can always ask for another session. I work for myself, and do not do third party payments, but rather operate on a cash basis.

Nor do I look at the clock: the sessions are always open-ended and usually last about 90 minutes, or until they reach a "natural" ending point. I have always been bothered by the practice of limiting therapeutic sessions to particular time limits. Somehow, back in the days of Freud and psychoanalysis and therapists depending on their making their living doing therapy, the "tradition" of the 50-minute hour became the norm for seeing a client. This means that somewhere in the room there is a clock that you can see unobtrusively (otherwise, how do you know when to start winding down a session and actually ending it?)! The odd thought hit me now as to how this would work if this is the way a surgeon carried out an operation like a hip or knee replacement?

After I look at the intake sheet[4] and ask about concerns, we "chat" with each other. I find out what has been bothering them, how long this has lasted, and what they would like out of this session. I certainly understand the constraints that exist both in private practice and institutional ones, yet I am fortunate to able to function without part of my mind always on the clock and how to end a session. This is probably why I also frown upon approaches which prescribe lists of steps to follow, i.e., what if your client balks at responding appropriately to step 4? What do you do next?

The main idea in the chatting approach is to connect with each other in this isolated room. I may tell stories, I may share some relevant personal information, and I may suggest an exercise like the Miracle Question or ambiguous function assignments or something else. [Having mentioned these two approaches here, I will briefly describe them at the end of this chapter, and also provide references to them.] The goal here is *being comfortable* with each other for this short period of time in which we will both learn some things about each other in the process of guiding them to discover realistic choices in their life.

For me, an exception in numbered approaches is Ernest L. Rossi's "moving hands" or " mirroring hands" four-step model, which is also an excellent example of a chatting approach (Hill and Rossi, 2017) which I sometimes use. The four steps are:

1 Holding your hands comfortably out in front of you and six to eight inches apart, will you find those hands somehow moving closer together as you think about what it is you would like to work on today, what you would like to change?
2 Now, will you find one of your hands (and arm) slowly moving downward as you review internally all of the relevant factors concerning that issue?
3 And now, will you find the other hand (and arm) slowly and easily moving downward as you think about several realistic ways of satisfactorily changing, that is, resolving those issues?
4 Finally, will you find your head nodding "yes" all by itself to let you know that you will be choosing and carrying out one (or more) of those ways? Thank you.

This is about as simple an approach as you can get in terms of: (1) what are you willing to work on and change today?; (2) explore your own relevant personal history with regard to what is concerning you; (3) find realistic solutions and actions—which *you* generate; and (4) kinesthetically ratifying that you will actually carry out one or more of those actions.

Rossi's moving/mirroring hands is only one of the ways with which I guide my clients into testing and experimenting to resolve their presenting concerns. (Please note that I use words like "bother" and "concern" and "trouble" rather than "problem.") In this book you will find a host of such approaches.

Thus, chatting involves two people spending time together while they explore together possible changes in the life of one of them. This does not involve taking detailed histories, and frequently involves methods which can be characterized as "secret therapy" in the sense that the therapist is not aware of much or most of the details of the client's concerns. It, of course, involves empathy, good rapport, attentiveness, observation, and total concentration. I am sure you may have other descriptions of this way of working, and most likely are already functioning in this manner in your own way.

D. The Fifty-Minute Hour

This book (subtitled "A Collection of True Psychoanalytic Tales") by the prominent psychoanalyst Robert Lindner (1955) contains five fascinating case histories. They are all worth reading, but the fifth one entitled "The Jet-Propelled Couch" (pp. 156–207) is the one that captivated me, and has remained in my memory for decades since it embodies an amazing principle of psychotherapy. The tale starts with a referral by another therapist of a key member of a secret security project of the government that stated,

> The fellow I am calling about is a man in his thirties, a research physicist with us out here. As far as I can tell he is perfectly normal in every way except for a lot of crazy ideas about living part of the time in another world—on another planet. Maybe this isn't so bad, but the trouble is he's really "gone" so much—if you know what I mean—that his efficiency is way below par and the operation here is suffering because of it. As I say, he's a physicist. Washington sent him out to do a key job, and until a few weeks ago he was going great guns. But lately he's out of contact so much and for so long that something's got to be done about it.

So, the physicist named Kirk in the book is shipped to Baltimore where he enters into daily sessions with Lindner.

This went on for many weeks with Kirk regaling Lindner with details of his fantasy world. Kirk drew charts of the galaxy where he was which was full of planets, and details about the main planet. Kirk was a good story-teller, and the details of his science fiction-like world made for fascinating listening to Lindner. Here are parts of the critical dialogue on p. 205:

K: About all of the stuff I've been giving you these past few weeks. It's all a lie, all of it. I've been making it up ... inventing all that—that nonsense!

L: You've been making it all up?

K: Yes. All of it.

L: It's all false?

K: All false!

L: Even the ... trips?

K: Trips! What trips? Why it's been weeks since I gave up that foolishness.

L: But, you've been telling me ...

K: I know what I've been telling you. But, believe me, I've been pretending for a long time. There've been no trips. I saw through all of the stuff weeks ago.

L: What do you mean, you saw through?

K: Just what I said. I realized I was crazy. I realized I've been deluding myself for years; that there never had been any "trips," that is was all just—just insanity.

L: Then why did you pretend? Why did you just keep on telling me ...?

K: Because I felt I had to. Because I *felt you wanted me to.*

About this dialogue Lindner comments (p. 206),

> Kirk was not able to appreciate the fact that when he abandoned his psychosis he had achieved my sole object for him: that to wean him away from his madness had been the conscious aim of my actions, and that this alone was important to me. As he saw and felt it, there had been a complete turnabout in our positions, a turnabout that confused and worried him, and one before which he felt helpless.

At this point Lindner was able to help Kirk get solidly back on his feet and go back to work.

One of the messages I drew out of *The Fifty-Minute Hour* is perhaps not completely justified by this tale: I state it as, "In any two-person interaction only one person can be crazy at a time." If this is true, then if you act crazier than your client he/she has no place to go to other than sanity! Certainly, being unpredictable can be shocking and confusing and works towards change and opens unusual and unexpected possibilities.

As an interesting coincidence here I am currently reading Zeig's book (2017, pp. 86–87) entitled *The Anatomy of Experiential Impact Through Ericksonian Psychotherapy.* On the cited pages is a description of a teaching session by

Carl Whitaker, the renowned family therapist. Whitaker was demonstrating working with a family who were sitting in an inner circle surrounded by an outer circle of students. During this session Whitaker fell briefly asleep three times. "The third time Whitaker fell asleep and awoke, the patient's father asked Whitaker to explain. Whitaker admitted, 'I often fall asleep when I feel anxious.'" This admission allowed family members who were initially anxious to feel more at ease. The psychotic young man, who was the identified patient, began to speak comprehensibly. The session ended favorably. Responding to a student's query Whitaker explained what happened as, "Craziness only occupies one space in a social system." An amazing illustration of the "Jet-Propelled Couch!"

In his own way, the late Frank Farrelly (the developer of Provocative Therapy (1974)) presented a startling way of doing therapy. I am not taking the space here to do a detailed presentation of provocative therapy, but just to cite its two central hypotheses (p. 52), followed by a number of thought-provoking (!) statements from his book. [As a caution, let me state that using provocative therapy requires studying the approach, skill, and practice. When I am stuck with a client, this is one of the approaches I frequently use.]

Hypothesis 1: If provoked by the therapist (humorously, perceptively, and within the client's own internal frame of reference), the client will tend to move in the *opposite* direction from the therapist's definition of the client as a person. [Emphasis added]

Hypothesis 2: If urged provocatively by the therapist (humorously and perceptively) to continue his self-defeating, deviant behaviors, the client will engage in self- and other enhancing behaviors more closely approximating the societal norm.

Thought-provoking statements (on pp. 36–48):

- People change and grow in response to challenge.
- Clients can change if they choose.
- Clients have far more potential for achieving adaptive, productive, and socialized modes of living than they or most clinicians assume.
- The psychological fragility of patients is vastly overrated both by themselves and others.
- The client's maladaptive, unproductive, antisocial attitudes and behaviors can be drastically altered whatever the degree of severity or chronicity.
- Adult or current experiences are as at least if not more significant than childhood or previous experiences in shaping client values, operational attitudes, and behaviors.
- The client's behavior with the therapist is a relatively accurate reflection of his habitual patterns of social and interpersonal relationships.

- People make sense; the human animal is exquisitely logical and understandable.
- The expression of therapeutic hate and joyful sadism toward clients can markedly benefit the client. [Farrelly's faith and experience.]

As an after-thought in this section, let me just recommend the books by R. D. Laing as a writer and therapist of yore whose writings continue to challenge the reader. As a sample, just dip into the slim volume of his poetry entitled *Knots* (1970). His poems and their confusing and pointed language force people to decide who they are and where they stand and challenge them in a similar way to Farrelly's work. They are fascinating reading.

1.6 Brief Introduction to Two Approaches

A. The Miracle Question and the Miracle Method

I believe that the use of the Miracle Question began with a client of Insoo Kim Berg of the Brief Family Therapy Center of Milwaukee (BFTCM). As I recall, she had a client who was stuck (as Insoo was, too) who said something like, "You know, if a miracle occurred, I could easily get over this." A "light bulb" lit in Insoo's head and she followed up by posing the Miracle Question to her client, and it worked. She and Scott D. Miller published a book about using this method as a radically new approach to working with problem drinkers in 1995.

Before discussing the Miracle Question it will be useful to summarize here the principles of the Solution-Focused approach, which was also pioneered at the BFTCM (Miller & Berg, 1995, p. 31):

1 No single approach works for everyone.
2 There are many possible solutions.
3 The solution and the problem are not necessarily related.
4 The simplest and least invasive approach is frequently the best medicine.
5 People can and do get better quickly.
6 Change is happening all the time.
7 Focus on the strengths and resources rather than weaknesses and deficits.
8 Focus on the future rather than the past.

Much has been written about this approach, and spending time studying it is useful. I recall a comment I heard Steve de Shazer make several times (and publish) about the solution-focused approach which went something like, "Would you rather spend your time listening to your clients talk endlessly about their problems and miseries, or about recent times when they were functioning well and free of constraints?" [Remember that, for whatever reasons, people do like to talk about their troubles!]

Since it is common now to always consult the web, I just did so about the Miracle Question and found many resources you can access. However, at this time I am just going to quote the Miracle Question as formulated by Miller and Berg (1995, p. 38):

> Suppose tonight, after you got to bed and fall asleep, while you are sleeping, a miracle occurs. The miracle is that the problem or problems you are struggling with are solved! Just like that! Since you are sleeping, however, you don't know that the miracle has happened. You sleep right through the whole event. When you wake up tomorrow morning, *what would be some of the first things* that would notice that would be different and that would tell you that the miracle has occurred and that your problem is solved?

I have a slightly different version of the Miracle Question, to wit:

> Just imagine that tonight while you are asleep that a miracle occurs. And this miracle is that *somehow* what you have come to talk to me about today is *fully and realistically* resolved. Remember that this is a miracle. So, tomorrow morning when you wake up, *post miracle*, what is the *first thing* you *will notice* that the miracle has *already* occurred?

Please notice that this is a shorter version of the Miracle Question and that I have italicized a number of key words and phrases. I precede this by saying (I may have said this earlier in the session),

> As you know my personal philosophy is that I always have hope and that I believe in miracles. I am going to ask you to think about something interesting at this time. If you are comfortable doing so, please close your eyes or look softly off into the distance.

These comments set the stage and expectation for the Miracle Question. Since I want my client to go "inside," I *suggest* that they close their eyes to remove all visual distractions.

Then I guide the client through the rest of their day with a series of questions asking them about how their day (and life!) *will be* post miracle. This is perhaps the most important part since I am guiding them to state out loud all of the different ways their life *will have changed* post miracle. They know much more than I do about their daily life and the changes that can realistically occur. As they tell me about these changes they are, of course, also telling and describing to themselves what these changes are. The more *detail* you can elicit at this time, the better. While they are telling you about these changes in their life post-miracle, they are, in effect, living those changes, they become *reified*. In a way, the Miracle Question is an example of an as-if procedure where they are telling you what will happen *as-if* it had already occurred. I hope you will notice how important it is to use appropriate expectational language here. Generally, this entire procedure lasts 15–30 minutes, and this depends on how skillful you are in asking about changes post-miracle, and how much the client responds.

Miller and Berg (1995, p. 43) give the following questions and I cite them as additional guidance:

- If the miracle happened, would that make a difference for you?
- What will you notice different about yourself when the miracle happens?
- What will others (spouse, family, friends, children, employer) notice different about you when the miracle happens?
- What difference will it make in your life when the miracle happens?
- What will you be able to do after the miracle happens that you could not do before?

While I think of it, I frequently use this question at appropriate points in the post miracle queries, "Now, just step outside yourself, perhaps to the front or side or back, and notice just what is different in how you stand and move and react post miracle." This dissociation step lets the person *observe themselves* from different perspectives, i.e., to see themselves from outside in this AS-If exercise.

B. Ambiguous Function Assignments (AFA)

Milton Erickson, in his inimitable way, got clients to carry out ambiguous function assignments (he pioneered this). These are suggestions for activities that are made to clients that are ambiguous in the sense that they do not appear to have a specific purpose. That is, the therapist implies (and expects) that when the client carries out this particular assignment that the client will learn something useful. Perhaps the most complete description of AFA is found in the work of Lankton and Lankton (1986, pp. 136–152). An AFA is, in effect, a second-order change (see Watzlawick, Weakland, and Fisch, 1974, pp. 10–11 and their chapter on this subject pp. 77–91 for details[5]). The Lanktons list 13 reasons for using AFA, and I think the main reason is that they work as second-order change, and primarily via the therapist's expectation (really, the placebo effect) that the client will discover during the AFA their own realistic ways to change. An authority figure (the therapist) suggests to them that they carry out one of the following AFAs given here as some examples of ones Erickson used as well as other possibilities.

1 One of Erickson's favorite AFAs was to suggest that his client climb Squaw Peak[6] in Phoenix, and then come back and report to him what they thought about on that hike. This can be generalized to climbing anything, including a hill or going up and down flights of stairs.
2 In Phoenix Erickson also suggested to clients that they visit the Desert Botanical Garden and the Heard Museum (Wonderful Native American collection) as AFAs.
3 Visiting any of the following and reporting back are good: museums (art, natural history, science, historical, aerospace, anthropological, ethnic, holocaust); zoos; national parks; a circus; and tourist sites.
4 Randomly opening one of the following and reading whatever is on that page and reporting back: the Bible, a dictionary, an encyclopedia, a biography, a classical novel, a children's story, a newspaper, a news magazine, a "how to" book of interest to the client, an anatomy book, a medical symptom book, etc.
5 Spending 30 minutes in a public place and carefully observing people (without staring!). Shopping malls, department stores, airports and other transportation terminals, zoos, downtown areas, concert halls, religious buildings, and parks are all possible locations for this exercise.
6 Carrying an object for a given period of time like a heavy stone around their neighborhood works. A variant of this is to go on a hike with a collection of stones in your pack and either bringing them back or discarding some along the way to lighten the pack.
7 Writing a letter to an iconic figure like God, Santa Claus, a guru, a historical figure or a fictional character and telling them what you need to lead a satisfying life, and that you just wanted to share this with them. (As a follow-up you could then write a letter to yourself imagining how they would respond!)
8 One final AFA is to pick a symptom that you wish to know more about or to change, and then do it in different place/way/duration. Then wonder how has this changed you and/or the symptom. (A classical AFA for couples is to change the side of bed on which they normally sleep!)

Basically, the object of doing an AFA is to get the client to do something that is generally out of the ordinary, and then to *wonder* about the significance of that activity (which they will then report back to you). The critical and effective part of AFAs is the therapist's expectation that their client *will discover* something realistically useful, and that reframes or changes their perspective. Again, you need to "hook" your client into carrying out an AFA!

Notes

1   This is a superb book and I cannot help but quote here four of the cover blurbs by distinguished professionals. Nicholas A. Cummings: "This is absolutely and unequivocally essential reading. It is perhaps the most comprehensive history in the development of practicing psychology by one of the giants who not only lived and developed it, but who best describes it. There are no other books that rival this book in its therapeutic relevance and comprehensiveness." Moshe Talmon: "Michael is one of the most versatile, integrative and creative therapists of our time. In this collection you will meet his mind, heart, and actions beautifully synchronized. This is a great book—don't miss it!" Bill O'Hanlon: "Brief Therapy and Beyond is an extraordinary tour de force. Strongly recommended." Michelle Ritterman: "Hoyt's magnum opus is delicious: erudite, literate, funny, and wise—a practical guide to the magic of rapid therapeutic rapport and change. How he knows all this is a mystery. There is nothing like it. Highly recommended."

2   In regard to the material in this section the reader may be interested in my book on healing language (Battino 2010).

3   This also applies, of course, to "majorities" depending on your ethnic and cultural and national and religious background. It is important to be aware of societal prejudices and historical segregation and discrimination.

4   Here I just list the items on my intake sheet: My name and address; Name, Phones; Address; Age, Birthday; Email address; Siblings (age and sex); Marital status; Children (age and name); Parents living? Ages; Brought up: rural, urban, suburban; Occupation; and finally—A *brief* statement of concern(s), and what you want out of counseling. This takes a short time to complete, especially since I do not have to eventually make a diagnosis that would satisfy an insurance company!

5   A first-order change is change within the system itself and is characterized by doing more of the same. A second-order change is *change of change* and is external to the system. Thus, a second-order change usually appears weird, unexpected, and nonsensical, i.e., there is a paradoxical element in the process of change.

6   The current name is Piestera Peak. It is the second highest peak in the Phoenix mountains at 2610 ft, and takes about 60 minutes to ascend with an elevation gain of 1208 ft, and 40 to return. I have done this twice, and the 360°views from the top are spectacular.

2   The Charlie Brown Exceptional Patient and Caregiver Group of Yellow Springs

morning angel light
a small irradiated cloud
we all watch and wait

2.1 Charlie Brown Group

Bernie Siegel founded a group called Exceptional Cancer Patients (ECaP) over 40 years ago. He was a surgeon in New Haven who had a lot of cancer patients, and found that one of the things that was missing in his practice was talking with his patients and their families individually, and in group settings. Bernie (he preferred being called by his first name) was a wonderful speaker and I had the opportunity to attend a number of his talks, attend a week-end of training in New Haven, listening to the many healing tapes he made, and also to correspond with him. After I read his first book (Siegel, 1986) I decided that I needed to get involved with an ECaP group and do volunteer work with people who had cancer and other life-challenging diseases.[1] I discovered that there was an ECaP group in Dayton that was meeting at Hospice of Dayton on the first and third Thursdays of every month. (In the early days of this group when there was a month with a fifth Thursday they generally had a guest speaker.) They kindly let me be an observer and attend their meetings.

The group was founded by Charlie Flynn, a hospice patient, two of his nurses, and a psychologist. It was named after Charlie and Dr. Brown who was his personal doctor. Charlie did the remarkable thing of "graduating" from hospice after he read Bernie's first book, and he decided he was not going to die of cancer. (He died about three years later on Christmas Eve of a heart attack.) I joined the group a while after Charlie died. His legacy lived on, and the group continued to meet in Yellow Springs (where I live), and was sponsored by the local senior center. I eventually became one of the facilitators, and then took over the group when it closed shop in Dayton and moved to Yellow Springs.

A typical meeting lasts 90 minutes. The following comes from the information sheet we give to new members.

GROUND RULES
1. CONFIDENTIALITY
2. POSITIVE ATMOSPHERE
3. PARTICIPATION IS VOLUNTARY
4. SHARE YOUR OWN EXPERIENCES, UNDERSTANDINGS, etc.
5. AVOID INTERRUPTING ANOTHER'S SHARING
6. LISTEN ATTENTIVELY (NO cross-talk)
7. REMEMBER CONFIDENTIALITY

FORMAT OF MEETINGS
1. WELCOME, announcements, business items, pick up name tags.
2. Introduction of GROUP PURPOSE (if new members present).
3. BODY OF MEETING—Each person introduces themself, stating NAME, why here, and shares some part of his/her life story (struggle, diagnosis, fears, coping, healing), and/or whatever else they wish to say for as long as they wish. Duration of this part of the meeting is 45–60 minutes.
4. SHARING WITH EACH OTHER—About 15 to 20 minutes will be available when the members can share with each other—within the group setting—specific items that have come up during the body of the meeting, or general information which they wish to share. [Note: this was not part of the Dayton meetings, but was added when we moved to Yellow Springs at the urging of one of our members. It has turned out to be an useful part of each meeting.]
5. CLOSING: Meditation/Imagery in a circle holding hands with one of the facilitators leading a healing meditation. (ca. 5 minutes)
6. Optional: Conclude the Closing with the SERENITY PRAYER.
7. HUGS are encouraged! (The Dayton group had a "chief hugger.")
8. HUMOR is always welcome since laughter can be the "best medicine." [Note: when people learn about this support group they sometimes think that it will be (in the vernacular) a "piss and moan" group. We seriously care for each other, yet we always find ways to laugh together.]

Earlier (section 1.4), I wrote about the distinction between curing and healing. We have found over the years that the most important thing that the group does is to help its members *heal* via being in an environment where they *know they are being heard* and listened to. Since everything said at a meeting is confidential, members are free to really speak their minds and share their feelings. Over the years I have found that the members become an extended family for each other, and are able to share things that they are realistically cautious in sharing with family or loved ones, or friends. This is an important function since I have come across many people who really need to be careful about sharing what is going on in their illness, i.e., people can react in surprisingly different ways when they find out that you have cancer or another serious disease. When I was growing up in the Bronx a long time ago the word "cancer" was always whispered and usually avoided. We always caution new members of our group to not be disappointed when someone close to them who finds out about the disease stops talking to them or avoids them. And, it is useless to attempt to find out why an old friend or relative effectively disappears. Some people (for whatever personal reasons) cannot confront the idea of your having a life-challenging disease, and just walk away. On the other hand, we also tell new members that there will almost always be other people who end up becoming important in their lives. That, too, can be surprising. I live in a small village (about 4000 people) and on many occasions I have found that almost spontaneously support groups just appear. These support people will provide meals and transport and other services. Sometimes, it can take a village to …

Another helpful thing that happens in our group is that being in the presence of others who are facing serious life challenges helps "normalize" how they feel about themselves and the disease. For example, it is useful to know that everyone else in the group has had feelings of depression and helplessness and hopelessness. At the ECaP workshop I attended we were told that one of the most important questions you can ask someone with a serious diagnosis is, "Have you fallen apart yet?" I believe that many, if not most of us, have been taught to be brave and strong and stoic and not show feelings. There is a tendency for those who know us to be cheerful and optimistic. This makes it difficult to share the feelings of depression and despondency that can be done in confidence in the support group. On the other hand, we also share the motto of our group, which is, "You may have to believe the diagnosis, but you do not have to believe the prognosis." Remember that a diagnosis is based on tests, while a prognosis is an educated guess by a professional. There are always "error bars" on prognoses.

I share here my personal philosophy, which is, "I always have hope, and I believe in miracles." Hope opens up possibilities. It also marshals a person's immune system and healing capabilities. Despair does weaken the body's ability to heal and recover. With respect to miracles, I have known several people who have "graduated" from hospice and gone on to live much longer than the original prognosis.

Three of the people I have met in these support groups are worth citing in telling about how they have coped with cancer. One told me about how he responded to people asking him how he felt. He said he told them, "Oh, there are some things wrong with my body, but I'm okay." He also told me that he managed to keep the cancer in abeyance for a long time by imagining that there was a circle of cowboys riding around the cancer locations within his body and killing off the cancer cells with their six shooters. (He was very fond of reading western novels.) Another friend who had prostate cancer told me that he talked to his cancer every day and told it, "I don't mind you being there and sharing nutrition with you, but you need to know that if you kill me, you are also going to die." A young art teacher, who showed up at our meetings with her bald head painted with flowers by her students, told us about how the chemotherapy she was having was painful and difficult to tolerate. She was quite religious, and told us at a subsequent meeting that the recent round of chemotherapy was not bothering her at all. She noted that the color of the chemotherapy fluid was yellow, and she told herself that this fluid was a "golden" gift from God. That image caused all of the side effects to disappear! Your mind and what you think and feel about your disease can have a profound physical effect. (There will be more about this in the chapter on guided imagery.)

In the ECaP workshop we were told about the usefulness of the following four questions:

- Why me?
- Why now?
- Why do I have this particular disease?
- Why am I getting better or worse at this time?

The answers to these questions will give you a great deal of useful information about how this person thinks *and* feels about their disease. It is not unusual for someone with a diagnosis of cancer, let's say, to feel that there is a reason they got this particular cancer, and that it appeared at this time in their life. Bernie has written and talked about how the different cancers may be connected to events or things in a person's life. An example is that a person has stomach cancer because there are things they have not been able to "stomach." This kind of connection may be fanciful, yet if a person has such a belief it is useful to know since it may be possible to counter that belief by reframing or other psychotherapeutic approaches. Also, the last question is informative in terms of letting us know what is going on in their life at this particular time, and how they feel about it. Responses to these questions, of course, are idiosyncratic. They are also important links into the person's belief system and personal history.

2.2 Ira Byock's Statements and End-of-Life Issues

Ira Byock, who spent many years as a hospice doctor, and has been involved in end-of-life issues for a long time, wrote a book (2004) entitled, *The Four*

Things That Matter Most. A Book About Living. His book actually lists five things that are important for a person nearing death to communicate to significant people in their life. In the following list I have added a sixth as 3A:

1 I love you.
2 Please forgive me.
3 I forgive you.
3A I forgive myself.
4 Thank you.
5 Goodbye

Statement 5 is obviously delivered at an appropriate time. Byock's book contains much useful information, and is well-worth reading.

My wife and I have been interested in end-of-life issues for several years. We have been active members of a community study group called the End of Life Community Forum, which met monthly for about three years. The group had guest speakers talking about various topics. We have also been presenters at a number of meetings. (At one time I was the convener of the group.) Topics have included things like living wills, durable powers of attorney for health, green burials, POLST[2] and MOLST,[3] ending your own life, Voluntary Stopping Eating and Drinking (VSED), hospice and related services, dying assistance programs like those in some U.S. states like Washington, Oregon, and California, overseas dying with dignity programs, methods of implementing choice in dying, amongst many others.

My wife and I are members of Final Exit Network (www.finalexitnetwork. org), a group of volunteers who will provide information on ending your own life when it becomes unbearable. They, of course, cannot assist and only provide information. Wikipedia describes this organization as:

> Final Exit Network, Inc., is a nonprofit organization founded in 2004 for the purpose of serving as a resource to individuals seeking information and emotional support in committing suicide [now generally called "self-deliverance"] as a means to end suffering from chronically painful—though not necessarily terminal—illness.

If you are interested in these issues, there is a great deal of information online. [See Appendix B for much more information about end-of-life issues.]

2.3 Rabbi Hillel's Wisdom

I am closing this chapter with two sets of sayings by Rabbi Hillel who lived about 2100 years ago. For the first sayings, which are a set of three questions, it is said that in his old age the Rabbi was asked to share his wisdom. Here are his well-cited questions;

- If I am not for myself, who will be?
- If I am only for myself, what am I?
- If not now, when?

The first question speaks to the fact that it is of basic importance in that we take care of ourselves. If we do not do this, then we will not be able to also care for others. Since we do not live in isolation, then we have obligations to be involved with all of the other people with whom we interact. The second question is realistic in the sense that we each need to be aware that we do not live in isolation, but in various communities. Although it is not stated explicitly, I believe the second question also applies to our environment. The third question is the *action* one: if we do not act in a timely fashion, then that inaction is the same as ignoring our obligations to ourselves and others.

Rabbi Hillel summarized in four sentences a philosophy of life that makes eminent sense to me, and is a guide to living an active and full life:

- I get up.
- I walk.
- I fall down.
- Meanwhile, I keep dancing.

In many orthodox Jewish sects dancing is an essential and integrated part of their religious beliefs. Dancing implies joy and happiness and dedication and involvement. I am reminded of an old adage which goes, "You have to give the Old Guy with the Scythe a moving target." It may be even harder for this "Old Guy" to cut down a dancer than an observer or a standee! So, meanwhile, keep dancing ...

Notes

1 At some point I decided that talking about life-*threatening* diseases was threatening and caused distress. I then changed to life-*challenging* diseases since the word "challenge" implies hope and change and action.
2 POLST (Provider Orders for Life-Sustaining Treatment) is an approach to improving end-of-life care in the United States, encouraging providers to speak with patients and create specific medical orders to be honored by health care workers during a medical crisis. (Please check if your state has passed a law legalizing this program or the following one.)
3 Medical Orders for Life-Sustaining Treatment (MOLST) is a program designed to improve the quality of care patients receive at the end of life by translating patient goals for care and preferences into medical orders.

3 Preparation for Surgery
Two Approaches

> heavily mossed trunk
> in its leafy sepulcher
> midges dance a dirge

In this chapter two approaches are presented for preparing people for surgery. The first is based on using hypnosis, and the second is based on Remen's healing circle. Since Remen's healing circle can be adapted to other areas than preparation for surgery, these will also be presented.

3.1 Hypnosis and Preparation for Surgery

A. Introductory Comments

Surgery is a physically invasive procedure that has been used since ancient times to cure all sorts of physical ailments. In the American Civil War the main surgery performed was to amputate limbs, and this was done before useful anesthetics had been developed. In modern times we have the use of many different forms of anesthesia for surgery, and these are abetted by muscle relaxants and drugs to calm the patient, and also remove the memory of the surgery. It is particularly the case for older patients that there is some amount of memory loss and even mild dementias and disorientation that can apparently last a long time post-surgery. On the other hand, modern surgery is painless during the surgery and quite effective for all sorts of ailments. I know that my knee replacement some 12 years ago was both needed and effective. Still, many people are fearful of surgery, and hypnosis for preparation and post-op recovery can be quite helpful. In this section I give details on how I do this with clients. (Please note that most of the material in this section was written about in detail in Battino (2000).)

In part hypnosis for preparation for surgery is based on an extensive earlier literature on patients being able to hear what is going on in the operating room even under the surgical plane of anesthesia. This literature is referred to in the footnote below.[1] Please note that the cited literature is old since I have not been able to locate more current research papers on this subject. There is also a large literature on *anesthesia awareness*, which is about some patients (about 100 to 150 cases per year in the U.S.) who can feel pain during the surgery, and also recall hearing speech during the surgery.

There is also evidence that people in a semi-comatose or comatose state can hear and understand what is being said to them. This is why it is frequently recommended that when you are with such people that you make physical contact like holding a hand, and talk to them saying whatever you wish to share and communicate. I have done this with friends who were in the last stages of their lives.

B. Five Parts to the Hypnotic Session

There are five parts to the hypnotic session:

1   Induction and relaxation
2   Pre-operation time
3   During the operation
4   Post-operation recovery period
5   Returning home and to normal functioning.

These five parts will become evident in the transcript that follows of a typical hypnosis session with a client I will call Mary. In the initial preparatory meeting (typically 90 minutes, there is no charge for these sessions as they are part of my volunteer work) I obtain information about the person's experience with surgery and anesthetics. Have they had surgeries before with anesthesia, and how had they reacted to it? I also find out if they have ever experienced hypnosis, or have their own way to meditate and relax. Since part of this procedure involves a dissociation, it is also important to find out from the client what is a "safe haven" or special personal place where they feel safe and secure, and is for them a healing environment. This safe haven may be real or imaginary, and I always request a few details about it so I can incorporate them in the CD. I want to know about their anticipatory fears and expectations and how they have coped with surgery (or something similar) in the past. I also tell them that I have prepared many people in the past who have gone comfortably through their surgery, and experienced less pain in recovery along with a faster recovery. I might also mention that there is a significant literature for using hypnosis for pain control and preparation for surgery. Then, I suggest that it would be useful to have a practice session here in my office to get their feedback before I prepare a CD with the same information on it. This is usually done at a session that is two to three weeks before the surgery. It is suggested that they listen to the CD as often as they wish before the surgery. (Since I have made many such CDs I can have one ready a few days after a session.) The essential part of this preparation method is a *posthypnotic suggestion* that activates prior to the beginning of the surgery. The client picks the time to activate the hypnotic suggestions, i.e., they may do this when they leave home, enter the hospital, when they are being prepped for the surgery, etc. This gives them conscious control of their experience. Of course, the client is highly motivated towards having this succeed.

C. Preparation for Surgery Script

The following is a model that therapists can modify to match their style of working in this manner. In it the ellipses (...) indicate pauses in the narration. It is quite important to allow the listener to have time to absorb and process what is said, that is, pauses of varying lengths are critical to the success of a recording like this. In addition, although I have not marked them out, it should be evident that certain words and phrases are "marked" by pauses and intonation. Since there is a lot of information in the five sections a preparation CD is longer than the recommended length for "standard" guided imagery CDs of 15–20 minutes.

Mary's Preparation for Surgery Script

Hello, Mary, this is the special CD I said I would prepare for you so that you would be able to go through the upcoming surgery in comfort, and to recover quickly and easily. We'll start again with you just paying attention to your breathing, just letting each breath go in and out, easily, simply, and naturally. And, with each inhale, chest and belly softly rising. Then, with each exhale, all of those muscles just relaxing. Just one breath at a time ... one heartbeat at a time. Be sure that you are in a comfortable position, and where you will not be disturbed, ... that your head and neck are free and easy, your jaw loose ... and knowing that at any time you can move a little bit to be even more comfortable. This is your time now, with nothing at all to bother you or concern you, a special quiet relaxing time.

Mary, you can count your breaths, too. Perhaps just one, two, three ... and then back to one. Easily, comfortably, simply. Occasionally, a stray thought may wander through. Notice it, thank it for being there, and go back to this breath, and the next one. This heartbeat and ... And, you know, as you listen to my voice as it goes with you, you can adjust or alter or change the words so that you are hearing exactly what you need now, and later ... Your peaceful time ...

And, within your mind now you can just drift off to that special safe and secure place that is especially yours. I don't know whether it is real or imaginary, yet it is your own special place where you are safe and comfortable and protected. ... This breath, and the next one ... Enjoy being there, looking around the pine forest near where you live. Breathing in the odors of the pine trees, enjoying that special peace and quiet, the serenity. ... One breath at a time. The trees stretch upward toward the sky, and the ground around you is strewn with pine needles making a soft carpeting, and an occasional pine cone. A quiet place. There may be the sound of wind in the branches up high, or a bird singing, or an insect. ...

While you are there it may be the evening before the surgery, or that morning, or when you enter the hospital, or when you are in the prep room. ... You will know just when to pay attention to your breathing again, just one breath at a time, as you drift away to your pine forest. ... And yet, easily and simply, you will be able to respond to any questions from the staff, you will be able to respond appropriately, perhaps looking back from the pine forest. And, you will be able to assist them in any way that is needed ... from there ... They would probably be surprised if they knew just where you are now, wouldn't they? ... One part of your mind is easily dealing with all of these mechanical details, while another part is enjoying the pine needles and the pine quiet. There is just a stillness and quiet all around you. ...

And now, your other mind knows that you have been moved to the operating room ... while you continue to enjoy being in the peace and quiet of the pine forest, observing, breathing calmly and easily. Perhaps you respond to a comment or message from your surgeon or the anesthetist who calls you by name, I do not know who. ... All is quiet and calm within your body. You are strongly alive, and yet willing to assist the experienced and concerned and highly trained medical people who are all around you. ... This procedure is going to proceed competently and professionally and successfully and rapidly. ... For you, this is almost like looking at a clock, and seeing the hands moving surprisingly rapidly as you continue, in a way, to be somewhere over there in the pine forest in your own special healing place. ... Is that a bird you hear in the background, or just quiet rustling sounds? It is all so quiet and pleasant where you are. ...

And, Mary, you should know that the procedure is going rapidly and well. Thank you. And, Mary, you do know, do you not, that you will be recovering from this rapidly and easily, comfortably, simply, and faster than you could ever have imagined. Thank you. ... And, what is it that you now see over there high above the trees circling in the sky? What bird is that? Can you also see some of those bright white fluffy clouds above the tree tops? Continuing to breath automatically and easily. ... Yes. And yes. ...

Mary, you do know that you will be quite comfortable after this is over, do you not? You will be able to request any medications that you need to be even more relaxed and comfortable, even though you will need surprisingly few. ... Your body has already started its own healing processes, regenerating, rebuilding, reconstructing, energizing, pulling together, doing whatever it needs and knowing how to do it, automatically, and without any awareness on your part ... just as you breathe simply and easily and automatically ... and walk and move ... your mind and body know how to do these daily simple automatic things. Yes, and yes.

And, at this time, Mary, the procedure has been successfully completed, ... and you know that, do you not, somewhere deep inside you. All this time you have been under the care of competent, concerned, and caring medical professionals. From time to time you have received healing messages from them ... first saying your name, and then saying "Thank you." And, within your mind now, you say thank you to all of them. ... Just continue to enjoy being in your pine forest as they complete their work, and move you to the recovery room. ...

Before you know it, you are in that recovery room, slowly and easily and comfortably waking up to your surroundings. You respond easily and calmly and simply to any questions, and are aware of who is there. You are smiling, since you have already been through the surgery, and are at ease. You might even be chatting with a relative or friend. Quietly, easily, comfortably. Remembering your time in your pine forest, the trees, and pine needles, and the quiet. There are always some pine branches on the floor of the forest, and sometimes an old tree trunk. You get fascinated watching the play of the dappled sunlight, and shadows, and some of the small bushes that are growing nearby. Such a peaceful time, now.

And soon, you know, with that other part of your mind, that you are now in that regular hospital room. You are feeling quite calm and rested, perhaps a bit sleepy. You ask for whatever you need, as you need it, ... and you can sense within in you just how surprisingly rapidly you are healing and recovering. There may be little sensations of warmth or coolness or tingling, all indicating that this is over, and that the healing time is here. ... Your body knows exactly what to do to heal and recover rapidly, and comfortably, resting as you need it, moving easily, responding to the staff as they continue to do their recovery work with you. ... You may not be aware of just how your body is talking to you now, just letting you know how rapidly the healing and recovery are proceeding, one minute, one hour, one day. ... And soon you will be going home to familiar surroundings and odors and sounds and people. I don't know exactly when you will say goodbye to your pine forest, knowing that you can always return when you need to, when there is another quiet time. ...

And, you know, Mary that all of this has been going on within an awareness of comfort, calm, and peace, just simply and naturally. Then, at some point, you are back to your normal way of being and living, with its familiar pace and sense. ... Normal time, and being. You may even wonder, with some surprise, that you are home again ... You may recall entering the hospital and leaving it and know that somewhere in between you have been helped by caring and competent medical people. And, here you are, now. Almost like awakening from a pleasant dream ... yes, it is over, and you are home and recovering easily and comfortably. ... And, you know that along the way, you have enjoyed many comfortable and calm and interesting moments, just recalling here and there little bits of what went on. This is your time now. ...

Mary, you know that your mind is somewhat like a recorder so that any time you need to remember what is on this CD, you will be able to remember and experience that fully, as you need it and when you need it. You can play these ideas and words over and over as you need them in preparation, perhaps in wonderment, looking back at how easy and simple and fast all this has been. ... And, now, Mary when you know somewhere inside of yourself that it is now time to be fully conscious and aware of wherever you are, ... and whatever you are doing, will you now find yourself taking a deep breath or two, blinking your eyes, stretching a bit, and coming back to this room ... rested ... here and now? Mary, I want to thank you for your trust, your confidence, and letting me spend this time with you. Thank you. ... Yes and yes and yes ...

Although the transcript above contain many ellipses indicating pauses in the narrative, when I deliver one of these preparations for surgery (and other hypnotic interventions) there are many more pauses than indicated here. The listener needs time to process what you are saying, and add their own imagery and memories and ideas. (In other writings I call this "pause power.")

D. Letter to the Surgeon and Healing Statements

Mary's surgeon's cooperation also needs to be elicited considering the earlier material about the patient being able to hear sounds in the operating room during the surgery. We postulate that this is possible, and to that end send the following letter to Mary's surgeon for her to give to the surgeon at an appropriate time. The letter can be mailed or presented to the surgeon at a pre-surgery meeting. The surgeon needs to know that I have prepared Mary for surgery using hypnosis. We want his/her cooperation. So, this letter needs to be written on my letterhead with some information about my background and credentials. The letter contains information about the rationale for doing this work. It also establishes that the client has been doing preparatory work of a particular kind, and that the client has certain expectations of the medical staff. The statements mentioned in the letter for someone in the OR to say to the client during the surgery are printed on a 5×8-inch index card, and laminated so the card can be made sterile. If you decide to do this kind of work, please feel free to adapt the letter and the statements to your and your client's particular needs. The letter and statements follow (without my contact information):

Dr. Betty Williamson
Dayton, OH

Dear Dr. Williamson:

I am writing this letter on behalf of Mary M. She has consulted with me concerning her upcoming surgery on XYZ and the kinds of things I can do to assist her to get through the surgery in the most comfortable and healing manner. For the past forty plus years I have been working as the facilitator of support groups based on Dr. Bernie Siegel's writings for people who have life-challenging diseases, and for those who support them. (Dr. Siegel is the author of "Love, Medicine, & Miracles" among other books, and is the founder of ECaP (Exceptional Cancer Patients.))

I also do individual volunteer work with cancer patients and other patients, teaching them guided imagery for healing, relaxation methods, ways of resolving unfinished business in their lives, and preparing them for surgery and other medical interventions and treatments. As to my credentials, I am a Licensed Professional Clinical Counselor (LPCC) in Ohio, and also a National Board Certified Counselor. I have published ten books in the counseling area, contributed chapters to other books, been a Faculty member at various international meetings, and have done training and taught courses in these areas, including hypnosis. I received my degree in counseling in 1978. Please consult my web site for additional information.

There is much evidence that patients, even under the surgical plane of anesthesia, can hear what is said in an operating room. It is believed that if the surgeon (or a designated person in the OR) makes encouraging and healing comments directly to the patient during the surgery, that this has a beneficial effect on outcomes and recovery. This has been both my personal experience for my own surgeries, and the experience of the people I have prepared for surgery. To this end, you will find enclosed a brief set of directions and some simple statements that we hope you (or someone else in the OR) will say to Mary at appropriate times during the surgery. To be sure that Mary knows she is the one being addressed, the statements need to be prefaced with her name, and always ended with a "Thank you" so she knows the message is over.

By the time of the surgery I will have spent some time with Mary preparing her for the surgery and the recovery period. She will have a CD which I have prepared for her with suggestions which she will have listened to several times before the surgery. I am certainly willing to talk with you or your staff at any time about my preparation methods. Please note that I am experienced in using hypnosis and am the co-author of a standard book on hypnosis, "Ericksonian Approaches. A Comprehensive Manual."

Sincerely yours,
Rubin Battino, M.S., Mental Health Counseling
Licensed Professional Clinical Counselor (LPCC), Ohio
National Board Certified Counselor (NBCC)
Adjunct Professor, Human Services (Counseling), Wright Stare University
copy to: M. M.

Dear Dr. Williamson (or Designee):

Please make the following statements (and/or other relevant statements) to me at appropriate times during my surgery. So that I know you are talking to me, please preface each statement with my name, and end each statement with, "Thank you."

1. Mary—Please slow down (or stop) the bleeding where I am working. Thank you.
2. Mary—Please relax your muscles in this area. Thank you.
3. Mary—This is going very well. Thank you.
4. Mary—You will heal surprisingly quickly. Thank you.
5. Mary—You will be surprisingly comfortable and at ease after this. Thank you.
6. Mary—Your recovery will be very rapid. Thank you.

3.2 Remen's Circle of Healing and Related Circles

A. Remen's Circle of Healing for Preparation for Surgery

Remen's book (1996) entitled *Kitchen Table Wisdom* gives details (pp. 151–153) on a healing circle that is designed to prepare people for surgery or other medical interventions like chemotherapy or radiation treatments. She is the medical director of Commonweal (www.commonweal.org), a retreat center for service and research in health and human ecology. A group of a few family members and friends is convened for the sole purpose of preparing the person, generally a week or two in advance of the surgery. The central person brings along a small (about one inch diameter) polished flat stone that is symbolically important to him/her. This central person gives the stone to a person in the circle next to them. (*Navajo Talking Circle* rules apply—see following section 3.2B.) Then, the person holding the stone talks briefly about some traumatic or difficult or medical event in their life. The stone holder then describes what personal characteristics or actions helped them get through that stressful time. These characteristics can be things like: love, courage, prayer, belief in a divine being, faith, persistence, or inner strength. This brief tale is then followed by the statement, "I put *faith* into this stone so you may have it with you." and passes the stone on. Each person in the circle thus endows the stone with their special way of coping and surviving. At the end, the stone, which has been embedded with all of these personal gifts, is given to the central person. That person will tape the stone to a wrist or hand before the medical intervention, and the medical staff are informed about its sacred significance. It is generally useful to let the medical staff (like the surgeon) know in advance that this is being done. Remen has used this healing circle for many years, and has received positive feedback from both patients and medical personnel.

B. Variants on Remen's Circle of Healing

Remen's circle of healing can be applied in many circumstances and for many purposes. For example, it can be quite effective in small groups for people who have assembled for weight control, smoking cessation, substance addiction,[2] or depression, among many other physical and mental health concerns. In such groups the person who is hoping and planning, but having difficulty, on ceasing the unhealthy behavior or emotion chooses a small object that is significant to them to be passed around. This object would be something they could easily carry on their person in some way. As the object is held by each person in the group in turn, they briefly describe what personal characteristics and actions have helped them change their life course. They then say, e. g., "I put perseverance in this for you," and pass the object on to the next person. In NLP terms, the object becomes a *kinesthetic anchor* for all of the characteristics put into it. Kinesthetic anchors are powerful behavioral modification physical reminders of what has been embedded in them. (This is like Pavlovian conditioning. It simply means that *physical* reminders—touching and feeling—are quite effective. Having "solid" reminders like Catholic counting beads, worry stones, or tying a string around your finger are more powerful than verbal ones.) I have a supply of small polished stones, one of which my clients can select, to help them remember the changes and ideas that have occurred in a given session. These stones "anchor" the work of that session.

Please imagine that you are working with a psychotherapy support group of some kind and one of the members is stuck and needs help and the encouragement of the group and to learn about the ways that other members in the group have used to overcome particular difficulties in their lives. This also provides the member with other *choices* of how to function, and in ways desirable to them. You may also use a bowl of stones, and one of them is passed around with each member briefly describing what personal characteristics or actions helped them out of their stuck place. So, this is designed to focus on one member of the group, and facilitate change for that person.

When I do workshops I enlarge this procedure so that all of the attendees have the opportunity to learn new behaviors and possibilities for change from a small group of volunteers. I recently did this in a workshop in London where there were 120 people in attendance; most were primarily from a hypnosis training group. In these workshops I like to have as many people as possible personally experience the approach or method I am presenting. At the front of the group was a table that had a bowl of candies in it (rather than small polished stones since the organizers forgot about the stones and "sweets" were available!). Four volunteers came to the front of the room. Each in turn picked up a sweet, held it up for all to see, shared a difficult time in their life, told about what personal characteristics or other things helped them through that difficult time, and then said, "I put courage/love/faith/ learning/friendship/therapy/hypnosis, etc., in this sweet for all of you." The volunteers then put their individual sweets back into the bowl, stirred them up and each removed one. I picked one up, too. Then, the five of us held hands with the sweet in the right hand, and made hand contact with the people in the front row. Then I asked everyone there (if they were willing to do so) to join hands with those sitting next to them. So, *physically*, we were all *in contact* with other people in the room. At that point I did a group induction (asking first, of course, if they were willing to participate) and said something like:

Here we are all together now, in contact with each other, hand to hand. So, closing your eyes, or just looking off into the distance, breathing softly and easily, naturally, just one breath at a time ... With each inhale chest and belly softly rising, and with each exhale all of those muscles just relaxing. ... This breath and the next one. This heartbeat and the next one. ... And, within your minds now you can just drift off to some special safe and secure place that is especially yours ... enjoy being there. That's right. This breath and the next one. ...

Something special happened here this afternoon. These four volunteers have put into the sweets those things that helped them through a time of distress and trouble in their lives. They and I are holding some of those sweets which have absorbed from the ones around them all those special helping phenomena. Somehow, somehow, those successful change agents have now been transmitted—not only to each of us holding hands here in the front of the room—but also to all of you in this room via the hands you are holding, and which are holding yours,—and the sound vibrations in the air from my voice resonating in your ears—and moving throughout your minds and bodies. Yes, and Yes. We are all together now, sharing the knowledge in the sweets ... this has somehow been transmitted through the air, and through our hands, so that each of us now has access to these learnings, these ideas, these ways of being and changing. ...

So, we are together here now, hand in hand, heart to heart, mind to mind, and spirit to spirit. And, so, within our minds we thank these four for their gifts to us. ... When you are ready, please gently squeeze the hand that is holding yours and which you are holding, take a deep breath or two, perhaps blink your eyes, and come back to this room, here and now. Hugs are always in order ... Thank you.

I have done the same presentation with respect to grief and grieving. The volunteers each pick a stone, and then tell the group what helped them through a significant personal loss. The stones are stirred up, each volunteer picks a stone, and we all hold hands while I do another related group induction or meditation on this topic. Again, the above approach can be done in any size group, and about any difficulty or concern. In many ways experiencing something like the above in a group can be more effective than individual work. On the other hand, as I have mentioned, using solid kinesthetic anchors do work well in individual therapy. (See section 9.6 for more on the use of Remen's healing circle for psychotherapy.)

C. Rituals, Ceremonies, and the Navajo Talking Circle

Hammerschlag and Silverman (1997) have written a wonderful and practical book about rituals and ceremonies. They make an useful distinction between rituals and ceremonies. *Rituals* are more like habits since they are repetitive and become incorporated into daily living. For example, we have morning rituals in terms of the order in which we toilet, shower, dress, and breakfast. These are *routine* actions and generally do not have their origins in religious or spiritual practice.

Ceremonies, on the other hand, are those actions that have a connection to spiritual, sacred, or religious practices. They are *special* events. Getting married or engaged, graduating from school, celebrating birthdays or anniversaries, and being baptized or bar mitzvahed, are all singular events (even though they may appear at regular intervals). Ceremonies will typically incorporate the following elements:

- leader to facilitate
- specific goal
- significant or sacred object
- group of selected people
- particular site
- mutual respect and reverence
- special timing
- specific order of service or components.

As an example, a typical Western culture wedding will include a minister of some faith, a wedding contract, wedding rings, relatives and friends, a special setting, a particular order of service, a specific time and date, the ceremony itself, and a following celebration.

Ceremonies can be used in psychotherapy and to mark special events in treatments or in healing interactions. In working with people who have life-challenging diseases ceremonies can be devised with the person for special events such as: successfully completing a round of chemotherapy or radiation treatments; celebrating scan results that show a decrease in the cancers in the body; although rare, graduating from hospice; or a decision to forego any further treatments. A friend of mine did the latter by writing out her decision and the reasons for it, and then burning this in her support group. She then took the ashes, put them in a Ziploc bag and put it out in the trash from her home. Successfully completing any round of medications has been celebrated by burying the medication container in a back yard. Recovery from orthopedic procedures like mending broken bones or receiving an artificial knee or hip has been celebrated by donating the walker and cane to a support group or an organization like Goodwill or the Salvation Army. After cataract surgery old glasses are donated. These ceremonies are, of course, worked out with the person involved.

With respect to psychotherapy there are many opportunities for ceremonies. Successfully getting over any addiction or debilitating habit like OCD, obesity, smoking, depression, anorexia, alcoholism, and drug dependence all come to mind. Leaving a treatment center with a clean bill of mental health is cause for a ceremony. Completing any form of psychotherapy and having attained your desired outcome(s) is celebratory, and worthy of commemoration. The therapist and his/her client can have a delightful time exploring ceremonial possibilities, and I have been privy to such times. Narrative therapists (see White & Epston, 1990) give their clients a printed "diploma" (sometimes on parchment paper!) describing their accomplishments.

The *Navajo Talking Circle* (Hammerschlag & Silverman, 1997, pp. 145–151) incorporates the elements that are cited above for ceremonies. In Chapter 2 I wrote about the Charlie Brown Support Group. In essence, the way this group functions is along the lines of the Navajo Talking Circle. There is a person who is the focus of this kind of healing group. This person supplies a sacred object that is passed around the group. (For certain ceremonies this would be a pipe.) You may talk only when you are holding the object. The rules are:

- Whatever is said and shared in the circle is confidential and not repeated outside.
- Each person talks about their own personal experience, from their heart, and for as long as they wish.
- When they finish, the next person has the attention of the group.
- There is no cross-chatter, interruption, or commenting on what others have said.
- Everyone listens attentively and respectfully to whoever is speaking.
- Each person speaks only once.

The leader of the group explains the purpose of the meeting, and may also explain the significance of the sacred object. The rules above are good ones and may be adapted to many different kinds of support groups.

3.3 Some Concluding Comments

This chapter covered the preparation for surgery information, and two versions of Remen's healing circles. I have carried out the preparation for surgery quite a few times with excellent results for the surgical patients. It is certainly open to adapting to other procedures and circumstances. The healing circle method has many applications for group work for support groups, addiction groups, habit changing groups (like smoking and weight control) and psychotherapy groups. [Of course, it helps to have a jar of small polished stones!]

Notes

1 Pearson (1961), Cheek (1959, 1960a, 1960b, 1961, 1964, 1965, 1966, 1981), Rossi and Cheek (1998, pp. 113–130), Dubin and Shapiro (1974), Liu, Standen and Aitkenheed (1992), Clawson and Swede (1975), and Bank (1985).

2 I do not like the term "substance abuse" since the substance is not being abused, but the person addicted to the substance is essentially abusing their own bodies and minds. The term "substance addiction" would be more accurate.

4   Case Study I

Mary and Anxiety and Insomnia and
Shit and Einstein and ...

> morning crow call
> and the rain on the roof
> weeping away tears

Mary, 63, called for an appointment. I said I worked as a single-session therapist, and it was her choice to have additional sessions. I told her I used hypnosis where appropriate. My fee for an open-ended session is $50. The phone call planted seeds.

At the session, she listed her concerns: chronic insomnia, anxiety, and past traumas. We started with insomnia. She had visited many professionals, used various medications (which helped for a while), and slept well for five to seven years before insomnia slowly returned.

I asked a question, suggesting she just let it rattle around inside her head during the session: "What are you willing to change today?"

Thinking that guided imagery (GI) would suit her, I asked for three pieces of information: (1) Do you have a way of relaxing and calming yourself?—She just lets her mind go "limp"; (2) Do you have a place within you, real or imaginary, where you feel safe and secure?—She likes to float in the ocean about three feet below the surface, somehow breathing easily there; and (3) Do you have an idea about someone or something that will let you sleep easily, naturally, and without anxiety?—Mary chose Eileen, an author, who would comfort, guide her to sleep, and rid her of anxiety.

Mary sat in an overstuffed armchair in the lotus position. I started with her paying attention to her breathing, and she went "limp" inside. I suggested that she just drift to her special place just below the water, and continue breathing normally and easily. I had her sense that Eileen was nearby, drawing close, making contact with her head, shoulder, or arm.

Eileen is knowing and powerful. She was able via contact to adjust all of the mental and physical parts of Mary that needed to be changed, so Mary could sleep easily, and without stress or anxiety. Mary cried silently for a while. When Eileen had completed her work, she slowly faded away. I then said Mary's mind, like a recording device, allowed memory and recall of whatever happened in this session whenever she needed it.

I gently roused her, and then, having her permission, held her hand for a while. I asked Mary to choose a smooth, colored stone from my jar of stones, to keep with her to remind her of the changes that had happened. Mary left looking calmer and relieved.

Ten days later she requested another session. Mary's request this time was for help with insomnia, and in coaxing her heart to love. She said, "Anxiety messes up sleep. If I can love, anxiety will decrease." After the first session she could sleep all night. A few days later anxiety returned.

Mary had difficulties with her parents, her husband, and a minister who turned her from God. She could no longer talk to or trust God. I decided to use the Miracle Question. This worked briefly. I asked her if Eileen could help with this and she answered "No." What to do?

I supposed to her that she had some internal demon that controlled her behavior. That idea made sense to her. Were there times when she could resist that demon and tell it to go away and stop bothering her? She said, "No!" She could not get rid of all of that shit inside of her. There was no way that shitting and eliminating could get rid of that stuff, and she cited the "Law of Conservation of Matter." Shit is matter, and will not disappear.

Einstein came to the rescue! I said that his famous $E = mc^2$ equation shows that matter can be converted to an equivalent amount of energy. I pointed to the West, saying the sun did this all the time. It was losing mass and producing the energy that it radiated. All those stars that you see at night are converting matter into energy.

Mary loved this idea, and her face lit up with joy. Now, she told me, every time she shat she would be cleansing her body and eliminating matter, that it would result in releasing energy and love. Anxiety would just disappear along with the shit.

She said she was reading Viktor Frankl's *Man's Search for Meaning*. I told her that I had met Frankl and had written a biography of him in play form. I talked about finding meaning in life, and then told Minnie's story from LeShan's book on cancer (1990). LeShan learned, working with terminal cancer patients, that what really helped them was asking about their unfulfilled dreams, and finding ways that they could have some fulfillment. Minnie dreamed about ballet. LeShan brought her books and articles, and she became totally involved with the ballet. Mary beamed, saying she always wanted to dance ballet, and that she was an excellent dancer. With her knee problem, attending ballet class was out, but she could join a Tai Chi class where the movements are balletic. Yes!

Mary agreed that she could forgive her parents and her minister when she recognized that they were fallible. She would not divorce her husband due to their adult children's attachment to him.

I suggested that laughter would help her through the time with her husband. She could dissociate and float away, observe him, and note what was comical about him and the situation. She laughed, saying this was a good idea.

The session ended. After a brief hug, Mary left. She returned two weeks later, still with sleep concerns, her heart opening up, and crap disappearing.

A dialogue with an unreconciled part of her made sense to her. She spoke with both parts, learning from each, and their resolution freed her. She wanted to return to New Hampshire. I said, "Once you have grown up in New Hampshire, you will always be there." Her face lit up and she asked me to repeat that. I did.

It is amazing what changes can occur when you follow the client's lead. When one approach doesn't work, it's good to use another! I wonder what would happen in *your* life if you just had a good ...

Commentary by Eric Greenleaf PhD

The best brief therapy is like a tasting menu of dishes, offered to a hungry person, who is not quite sure ... Rubin Battino, with a scientist's observation and a poet's skill, brings dish after delicious dish to Mary's attention, until she is beaming with satisfaction. Imagery, hypnosis, Gestalt, metaphor, solution focus, relationship—a top chef can cook with any ingredients, and good digestion follows.

[Note: This case study was published in the *Milton H. Erickson Foundation Newsletter*, Vol. 38, No. 3, December 2018, p. 6.]

Commentary by RB

Mary was one of my most challenging clients. I thought at the end of the first two sessions that we had worked through all of the stuff that had been troubling her. In the third session a few more items showed up. The main one was primarily resolved via the Gestalt Therapy Two-Chair method. Mary got right into it, easily playing both parts and working out (for herself) what she needed. My off-hand comment about growing up in New Hampshire appeared to be right on. The main takeaway of this case study (as also noted by Greenleaf in his commentary) was my ability to keep changing modalities to find ones that worked for Mary in those particular sessions. I was a bit surprised that the Miracle Question did not work, but that the Narrative Therapy externalization one did. The de Shazer recommendation of, "If it isn't working, do something different," once again recommends itself!

5 Case Study 2
Bobbi and Her Needy Knees

> I opened my mind
> to the wind in the chimes
> tinkling tinkles

Bobbi is someone I've seen in sequential single-session therapy (2012, 2014, 2015, and 2018). She is 71 now and her opening comments (in 2018) were about: dementia in her family, arthritis issues, and a bike accident that did some damage to her right knee. She has a fascinating, challenging, and interesting job. She has been an active square- and line-dancer since 1978, has done demonstration dancing, has participated in large square dance meetings, and been a dance leader and teacher. Bobbi has been to a number of doctors, and her orthopedic doctor indicated that both of her knees had significant arthritis. Her doctor also said that for some unknown reason there was pain, discomfort, and difficulty only in her right knee even though they appeared to be in the same condition. Her expectation of this session was that she would be able to convince her head that her right knee was as good as her left knee (so she could continue to be active in dancing).

Where to start? I told her that I have an excellent orthopedic doctor (if she wanted a second opinion) who actually specializes in "revisions," that is, fixing other doctors' mistakes. I also told her that I had recently completed ten sessions of Rolfing (Structural Integration), which she might consider. I then mentioned having been in Feldenkrais workshops where we did certain movements and stretches on the right side of our body, and then imagined "transferring" the ability to do those movements to the left side of our body. All of the workshop participants experienced this kind of transfer: this seemed magical to us and, yet, possible because of mind/body interactions.

To emphasize this possibility I then told Bobbi about how Milton Erickson recovered most of his bodily movement capabilities after having polio as a teenager. (See my biography of Erickson for details of how he did this, Battino, 2007.) After being totally paralyzed and in a coma for several days, he discovered that the rocking chair he was strapped into moved when he wanted to get closer to a window. Erickson then realized that by mentally concentrating on the muscles needed for each movement in his body that he could actually contract those muscles. So, he in effect, was able to re-activate these wired-in and remembered movements. These stories were told to build the expectation and possibility of Bobbi being able to do the same thing.

For the next part I first thought of using the Gestalt Therapy "Two-Chair" approach and have Bobbi be her left knee in one chair and the right knee in the other, and then let the left knee teach the right knee how to be like it. This would have been awkward in the room we were in. So, I decided to use a variant of Rossi's "Moving Hands" (now called "Mirroring Hands," Hill & Rossi, 2017) approach in the following way. I had Bobbi sit with her feet about six inches apart, her left hand on her left knee, and her right hand back on her right thigh. Since Bobbi had experienced my hypnosis style and voice, I gave all of the following directions in that manner.

Your left hand is now receiving information from your knee about all of the necessary changes needed to decrease the pain in your right knee, and regenerate/reconstruct/rebuild and renew your right knee: cell by cell, tissue by tissue, ligament by ligament, nerve by nerve … slowly, easily, naturally, automatically. Just restoring it in surprising and interesting ways. That information is somehow already on its way up your arm and crossing through your shoulders and brain to its right side. You know that neural information will now be passing from the right side of your brain to the left side, easily and automatically. Gently remove your left hand from that knee and now place your right hand on your right knee.

I do not know just how you will sense this movement of information and ability to change and transform. There may be sensations of tingling or warmth. Yet, you do know, do you not, that your mind and body have remarkable powers and the ability to change and to rebuild, homeostatically. Now, recall in detail how your knees, and other parts of your body, were developed and formed and maintained? Slowly, easily, naturally … just let this information and needed changes begin to embed themselves in your right knee. We may not know exactly how these changes occur, yet, somehow, somehow, change and stability can and do occur. When you sense that this particular transforming transfer has occurred, move your right hand back and place your left hand back on your left knee.

This is just a beginning, is it not? And, at this time, even more effective changing rebuilding, and transforming neurological and physiological information has already begun to move from your left knee into that hand and is on its way upwards. When you sense that these extra and new change capabilities are on their way, slowly remove your left hand and move your right hand into place. Again, slowly, easily, naturally, comfortably, your right knee area is receiving and storing and processing and beginning to utilize, yes? Yes.

Continuing to breathe slowly easily, and naturally, there is one more thing to do. Just let your two hands come gently together. And, your right hand can simply thank your left hand, and all of the parts between your left and right knees, for this healing and transforming experience.

You should know that at this time in natural ways that will continue, your mind and body can and will continue this work. Also, you now know how to continue this work on your own for any other changes that are needed.

I want to thank you, Bobbi, for your trust and your confidence, and when you are ready, just take a deep breath or two, gently stretch, perhaps blink your eyes, and come back to this room here and now. Thank you.

After a short quiet time we also discussed how she could continue her dancing activities in appropriate ways. When Bobbi left she was smiling and moving easily.

I trust that the reader can find many occasions and ways to adapt this procedure. May I close with saying that this was a *moving* experience?

6　Guided Imagery for Healing and Psychotherapy

barely moving breeze
orange moon through the treetops
soft shining shadows

6.1 Introduction

Guided imagery for healing was started by Carl and Stephanie Simonton. He is an oncologist and she is a psychotherapist. They wondered how they could use imagery with cancer patients to guide them into using their own thoughts and feelings to influence body functioning, and its own healing capacities. So, they tested this with groups of cancer patients, getting them first to relax, and then introducing imagery that was designed to enhance body resources in removing cancer from their bodies. The initial emphasis was on imagery, and used the patients' imagining that there were sharks or wolves within their bodies that would seek out cancer cells and masses and gobble them up and destroy them. This originating work is described in Simonton et al. (1980). Also, see Simonton (1984). Initially, the healing imagery was chosen by the therapist. At some stage it was pointed out by some patients that they were uncomfortable with having wolves and sharks in their bodies! In doing individual work using guided imagery it is important to find out what healing imagery or entity will work for a particular client, that is, *let them make the choice.* When doing guided imagery with groups or making general guided imagery recordings on a particular subject, it is important to use permissive language so the listener can make his/her own choice. Not all listeners can easily visualize, so it is important to include both auditory and kinesthetic language in guided imagery. We use the word "imagery" in a general way that includes visual images as well as all of the other senses.

The formalism of guided imagery can also be used for psychotherapy. The basic approach is similar, the difference is that the healing modality or entity is one that helps/aids/guides the client through behavioral, emotional, attitudinal, and mental changes. There are overlaps with other psychotherapeutic approaches. This will be discussed in some detail later in this chapter.

6.2 Different Forms of Imagery

The detailed descriptions given here are based on those in Achterberg, Dossey, & Kolkmeier (1994). (Also see Achterberg (1985) for one of the pioneering books in this area.) *Receptive imagery* refers to those that are received in the moment rather than those that are created. They just pop up, and are more like those in dreams. They typically occur in the *hypnagogic* state (the in-between time when you are falling asleep) or the *hypnopompic* state (when you are waking or half-awake).

On the other hand, *active imagery* involves a conscious and deliberate effort to construct an image. This is volitional, and you can choose a specific image for eliminating cancer cells or healing an infection faster. This is a way of directly "speaking" to your body. It can be symbolic using metaphors, or realistic in terms of physiology. (Later in this book I will write about communicating more directly with your body via ideomotor signaling.) It is most important when doing individual work that you find out from your client what imagery they sense and feel would work for them.

To be a bit more specific, *concrete imagery* is the kind that is biologically correct imagery. One of my clients was a professor of biology, and always chose concrete imagery, which made more sense to him than metaphoric imagery. Most people select *symbolic imagery* for this kind of healing work. They feel, in terms of their own belief systems, that a religious figure or a guru, or healing touch or healing hands or a healing spirit, will be more powerful and effective. If, for you, a power animal is your choice you already have an image and a sense of that animal (which I do not). You always need to work within and utilize your client's belief systems and background and memories.

We can distinguish two more kinds of imagery. *Process imagery* is the mechanics of how an image works or is used, i.e., the steps for implementing the activity of the image. As an example, if the image has to do with eliminating lung cancer cells from the body using the comforting image of your father when you were ill as a child, you first need to call up his presence. (Your father may be alive at this time, or may have died.) Do you call him, or sense his presence near you, or reach out your hand for him to hold? Once he is present, you can give him instructions as to what you want him to say or do during this visit. Then, you might imagine that somehow from this contact he is transferring to you and your immune system the knowledge, power, and ability to easily and efficiently eliminate the lung cancer cells wherever they are within your body. Before this visualized contact is ended (gently) you can imagine him telling you that your immune system will continue to work effectively and efficiently since it has now learned how to eliminate and destroy those cancer cells. Also, you might add that he kisses and/or hugs you before leaving.

Another, and important, kind of imagery is *end-state imagery*. This imagery is of you in your healed state, that is, where the disease or condition has been completely eliminated, or eliminated to your satisfaction. In doing art therapy it is useful to ask the client to draw four pictures: (1) a drawing of you in your current physical condition; (2) a drawing of the treatment(s); (3) a drawing of you in your final healed state; and (4) in your judgment how you got from (1) to (3). So, end-state imagery is related to the "crystal ball" approach frequently used in psychotherapy where you ask the client to go into their future to the point where their troubles have been resolved, look back, and tell you what it was they did to get to that desired state. This is in the realm of acting "as-if" your life has already changed, and the more detail you can elicit about that end state, the more real it becomes. Hidden in here is both expectation and hope and lots of personal information that we as therapists do not generally know. That is, the client knows him/herself and his/her capabilities and potentials and history better than we do: end-state-imagery facilitates access to their own healing capabilities.

When you do guided imagery work, especially for groups, the images need to be general or generic. And, you need to be experienced in using these kinds of imagery. In such a setting, I generally give the audience a choice by a show of hands as to which of the following kinds of general imagery they would prefer me to use: (1) healing light or energy from a potent/powerful source; (2) healing touch, usually healing hands; (3) healing warmth or coolness; (4) a healing presence—either unspecified or a healing guru, wise person, outer or inner guide, guardian, or religious figure; (5) a journey or pilgrimage or trek to some healing object, person, or location; this may be to a healer, and it may involve receiving a healing object or ingesting a healing substance; and (6) being in the presence of a "power" animal or totem or fetish that has restorative or curative capabilities. Of course, it is possible (and not unusual) to combine several of these healing entities in one session. These need to be in your repertoire.

Perhaps, the best known person in the guided imagery field is Belleruth Naparstek. Her web site is www.healthjourneys.com and it lists her books (in the reference section), and many recordings on many many subjects. The recordings are all professionally done, and have specially designed music accompaniments. I recommend her three books, which are: *Your Sixth Sense: Unlocking the Power of Your Intuition* (2009); *Staying Well With Guided Imagery* (1995); and *Invisible Heroes: Survivors of Trauma and How They Heal* (2005). You may also wish to read the Wikipedia article on her and her work.

6.3 Duration of Guided Imagery Sessions

There are two main parts to guided imagery sessions: (1) orientation and relaxation; and (2) delivery of the guided imagery itself. In the first part relaxation is used for two reasons. The first is to establish a peaceful and calm time for the recipient. The second is that in the relaxed state the mind is more open to suggestions, and guided imagery is all about suggestions for healing. The deepest level of relaxation is generally reached in about ten minutes. However, we have found that only two to three minutes are needed for this at the beginning of the session since suggestions for continuing relaxation can be repeated throughout the delivery portion. It is recommended that a guided imagery session last between 15 and 20 minutes. Indeed, Naparstek's and Bernie Siegel's and my sessions are all within that time frame.

6.4 Information for a Guided Imagery Session

When I prepare a guided imagery recording for someone or do the first one for someone face to face, I ask for the following information:

- Do you have a preferred way of relaxing or meditating or doing self-hypnosis?[1] (I use the client's preference if given. Otherwise, I tell them that I will just use counting breaths or paying attention to breathing.)
- Do you have a personal " safe haven"? That is, a place within your mind that is real or imaginary where you go that is a safe and secure and healing place for you? Ask for a few details about that place.
- Do you have an internal sense or feeling or idea or image of what will work for you in healing and helping you at this time? Please give me some details about this healing/helping entity or modality. (If the person cannot think of anything at this time, I mention what others have chosen like healing hands or healing light or a healing religious figure.)

These personal preferences are incorporated into the session.

The session ends with the observation that,

> You know that your mind is somewhat like a record device so that you will remember what has been said so you can recall everything that is useful to you. Just find a quiet place where you will not be disturbed, pay attention to your breathing, and remember.

There is always a "Thank you" at the closing.

Sometimes it is useful to make physical contact with the client in the imagery portion of the session (always get permission for this beforehand). This is used to enhance the healing imagery. At that point I will say something like,

> Would it be okay to hold your hand now? [If, yes, reach out and gently hold their hand.] Somehow, somehow, from me and through me you will sense now that there is a special healing going on in just those parts of your body

where it is needed. You might even feel some warmth or coolness or tingling in those places. That's right. Easily and simply and automatically. And, your immune system is learning and becoming more effective, more efficient, more knowledgeable. It is almost as if every part of you has become stronger and healthier. Somehow, from me and through me.

(This will be detailed in one of the guided imagery transcripts to follow in this chapter.) In NLP terms the imagery is enhanced via a kinesthetic anchor. And, touching can be a quite powerful change agent.

6.5 Other Factors: Connections to Metaphor, Hypnosis, and Psychotherapy

Metaphors are stories that you tell to clients to engage them and to provide them with possibilities of responding differently in their lives. The metaphor generally *parallels* something in the client's life rather than matches existing actions and moods and feelings. If the plot and characters in the metaphor are too close to actual events, then the client may sense this and feel manipulated. The healing modalities and entities in a particular guided imagery, and the way they are presented, actually become metaphors for change. This is even the case when the imagery is physiologically accurate, i.e., requested by the client. The guided imagery portion of a session in effect *guides* the client on a special internal and fantasy journey.

My working definition of hypnosis is *focused attention*. Generally, during the delivery of the guided imagery the client closes his/her eyes and goes "inside." (Closing eyes is not necessary, and the client needs to be given permission to do so or not. "If you feel comfortable doing so, please close your eyes now, or just let them look off into the distance or be unfocused.") Another way of describing hypnosis is to consider that any time a person goes "inside" (their mind), they are in a hypnotic state. The "depth" of this state does not seem to matter. The "message" in guided imagery is in effect a *post-hypnotic suggestion* for certain changes to occur. That is, the expectation is that the healing modality or entity will actually bring about physical and/or mental changes post-session. That expectation is the post-hypnotic suggestion. In practice this means that it is useful (almost required) that the person delivering the guided imagery be trained in hypnosis. I know that my experience as a hypnotist enhances the guided imagery work that I do. The delivery in the entire guided imagery session benefits from knowledge about the usefulness of pauses, and highlighting particular words and phrases, for example.

Although the origins of guided imagery work lie in treating physical diseases like cancer, this approach can also be quite effective in psychotherapeutic practices. In my recent work, and certainly in some clinical demonstrations I have done, I found myself using guided imagery as the framework for the session. Somehow, I just naturally slid into that way of functioning. In the next two sections I am going to present a transcript of a guided imagery session for physical healing, and then one for psychotherapy. I do not have transcriptions of actual sessions or of the many CDs I have prepared. So, the following are recreations of past sessions, and are also syntheses of some of them. Each "transcript" has an introductory section.

6.6 George's Guided Imagery CD for Cancer

George is one of my oldest friends and had been recently diagnosed with third stage prostate cancer. This was one of the malignant types and not one of the benign ones that men can live with for a long time. George had done some meditating at one time, no longer practiced, and thought that paying attention to breathing was a good way to relax. His safe haven was a place in Jasper, Canada, on the island on Pyramid Lake facing Pyramid Mountain. It turned out that on one of our travels that my wife and I had actually visited Jasper and done a hike in the Pyramid Lake area, so I could easily describe that place. George had two healing images he wanted me to use: one was of a specific event when he was a teenager and was very sick. He recalled his father (with whom he was very close) sitting by his bed for long periods of time and holding his hand. George is Jewish and also felt that the healing presence of G*d or Hashem (since Jews do not say the name out loud) would get rid of the cancer or meliorate its progress and symptoms. I told George and others I've worked with who had life-challenging diseases that the guided imagery would help him, that miracles did occur, and that there were no guarantees. In the following, ellipses indicate pauses or varied lengths.

A. George and Pyramid Mountain and Hashem

Hello, George, this is the healing CD that I said I would prepare for you. Please be sure that you are in some comfortable position, and in a place where you will not be disturbed for the next 20 minutes or so. As I told you, I like to start out with your paying attention to your breathing. Just notice each breath as it comes in and goes out. Slowly, easily, naturally. And, with each inhale, chest and belly softly rising. And with each exhale, all of those muscles just relaxing. That's right, one breath at a time. One heart beat at a time. Occasionally, a stray thought may wander through. Just notice it, thank it for being there, and go back to this breath, and the next one. Just breathing comfortable and easily. And, if you need to move a bit to be more comfortable, please do that. One breath, one heart beat. Your healing time now, with nothing else to bother you.

And, within your mind now, just drift off to that wonderful safe healing place of yours, Pyramid Lake. You might imagine parking your car and walking down to the short bridge out to Pyramid Island. You may stop on the bridge and look out across the water rippling in a breeze, to the mountains beyond. And, then, you have reached the island and slowly walk along the path to the far side. Continuing to breath softly and easily. There is a bench there, and you sit down, looking across the water to Pyramid Mountain with its massive triangular shape rising up towards the clouds. An interesting visage with all of those rounded surfaces, variegated in color, just across the water. And, at water level and rising up are all of those evergreen trees framing the lower part. One breath at a time. With the wonderful odor of an evergreen forest. How many thousands and thousands of years ago did that mountain rise and get its shape? Your quiet and restful healing place. Enjoy being there.

And, while you are there, your mind drifts back to a time when you were a teenager and in bed and your father was sitting beside you. That was a difficult and maybe a scary time back then. And, your father was holding your hand and staying with you, and talking softly to you. He may even have been telling you a favorite story, or describing a time you were fishing together. This breath and ... That was then, and now, an inner sense of safety and security and peace are with you. You knew then that you would get better. There is nothing like a parent's unconditional love to protect and heal you. What a wonder ...

And, now, while you continue to feel and sense your father's being with you, holding your hand, something interesting happens. You sense someone, someone special, coming closer to you. A powerful and knowledgeable healing presence. I do not know exactly how Hashem appears and comes to you at this time. Yet, you know that He is there with you, reaching out his healing love and strength and power. And, you can almost feel Him lightly touching you, perhaps on your head or an arm. And, Hashem knows just exactly where within your body to send His healing knowledge, His healing power. Just strengthening your immune system and making it more effective, more efficient, more knowledgeable, more capable of guiding your body to eliminate those crazy cells, just as fast as your body can get rid of the detritus. Slowly, easily, naturally. And, Hashem's healing touch is continuing to work. You can almost sense, can you not, that somehow, somehow, almost cell by cell and tissue by tissue and nerve by nerve, these changes are occurring? One breath at a time. Breathing softly and easily, enjoying being at Pyramid Lake, feeling your father's healing hand, Yes, and Yes, and Yes.

Hashem has more work to do and more people to help and heal, and slowly moves away. Leaving within you a stronger, more effective, more powerful immune system. Strengthening all of your body's healing systems. And, within your mind now, you thank Hashem for this gift and His love. You also thank your father for his love and his gifts and his faith in you.

And, you know George, that your mind is somewhat like a recorder, so that you will be able to recall and remember what has been said, and all of your feelings during this time. Whenever you need to refresh these feelings and memories, all you need to do is find a quiet place, pay attention to your breathing, and remember. So naturally ...

I want to thank you, George, for your trust and your attention and your love. And, you know that I love you. Many, many years together. And, when you are ready, please take a deep breath or two, blink your eyes, stretch a bit, and come back to this room, here and now. Yes and Yes and Yes—thank you.

With appropriate pauses and emphasis on various words and phrases this is an example of a healing CD. The recording would be about 15 minutes long. People are instructed to listen to it as often as they wish. Generally, there is just one healing modality or entity—George had asked specifically for the two in the above guided imagery session. There is one other recording that both George and his wife found to be useful and that is my sleep and relaxation CD, which has me using my quiet hypnosis-oriented delivery for about 30 minutes. Recall that I make a distinction between healing and curing. This was a healing CD designed to provide comfort, relaxation and hope. Sometimes a guided imagery CD will result in a cure for the disease, and sometimes a prolongation of life. However, there are no guarantees. My personal philosophy is that I always have hope and that I believe in miracles. In terms of the latter, I have known several people who have had extended lives beyond medical prognoses, and several other people who have "graduated" from hospice programs. My expectation is that these CDs will heal.

6.7 Anne's Guided Imagery for Psychotherapy

Anne is a 48-year-old psychotherapist. She lives and works in the small (ca. 4000 population) college town in which I also live. Paying attention to breathing is relaxing. She has done some yoga. Her safe haven is the pine forest in our local forest preserve. Anne is quite religious and her chosen healer/helpers are Jesus and the Holy Spirit. She came to see me since she has had occasional deep anxiety, which began about six months ago. Before I started the guided imagery session I asked her permission to hold her hand sometime during the session. She said that this was okay.

A. Anne and Anxiety and the Pine Forest and Jesus

Anne, please make yourself comfortable in that chair. If you need to move at any time to become more comfortable, please do so. And, we can start with you just paying attention to your breathing, noticing each breath as it goes in and goes out. With each inhale, chest and belly softly rising. And then with each exhale, all of those muscles just relaxing. You can imagine that each inhale is a kind of energizing and healing breath; and that each exhale is a cleansing and clearing breath. Just one breath at a time, one heartbeat at a time. Slowly, easily, naturally. Occasionally, a stray thought may wander through your mind. Notice it, thank it for being there, and just go back to this breath, and the next one. That's right, comfortably and naturally. This is a peaceful time for you now, a calm one, and there will be nothing to trouble you, just sitting there at your ease. Another easing breath, and this heartbeat. Enjoy this time.

And, within your mind now, just drift off to the Pine Forest. Walking through the woods, along the trail. Perhaps a soft breeze is moving in the tree tops. Maybe a bird singing above, you touch the bark of a tree, and feel the ground underfoot. And, as you walk along, there is the creek running by you. Take in a deep breath, look at the running water, see the ripples and the stones underneath. Yes. And, then it is up through the woods to the entrance to the pine forest. The tall trees, the bushes underneath, a soft bed of pine needles, that aroma of pine forest. An amazing peacefulness and quiet surrounds you. In the center there are some fallen old tree trunks. You sit on one, quietly enjoying being surrounded, protected, by all of those old evergreens. Yes, ever green, a marvel.

And, while you are there, something interesting happens. Your eyes may be closed now, and yet you sense the presence of someone, something holy, a spiritual place, almost like being in one of those ancient cathedrals. And, the pine forest is somewhat like a natural cathedral, is it not? The Holy Spirit comes closer to you, close enough to reach out and perhaps touch your head or arm or shoulder. That contact is gentle and, yet, almost electric. The Holy Spirit is a healer and through its touch it is sending peace and quiet and calm into every part of your body. Almost as if each atom, each molecule, each cell, each tissue and bone and nerve, is being anointed with a healing and calm energy. I do not know where within you you are feeling this transformation, these changes. There might be a tingling here or there, or a bit of warmth, or a sense of being touched ever so gently and lovingly. The Holy Spirit knows just where to send and incorporate this sense of peace and calm, does it not? Yes and Yes and Yes.

Would it be okay now to reach out and hold your hand? I note that your hand is not moving and that is fine. For you are now in the hands of the Holy Spirit, and perhaps Jesus, too. There is that peace that somehow seems to go beyond, and out there, to perhaps somewhere out in the heavens. Yes and Yes. Continuing to breathe calmly and easily and naturally. This heartbeat and the next one. They have reached out to you and touched you, and now it is time for them to move on for they have more healing work to do. Within your mind now, you thank them for their healing love and presence, for you know that they will be with you as you need them and when you need them. Your peaceful time now.

And, within your mind now you can rise and say goodbye to the pine forest, and gently wend your way home. Enjoy this quiet walk through the woods. Yes.

I want to thank you Anne for your attention and your trust and your confidence. And, now, taking a deep breath or two, blinking your eyes, and maybe stretching a bit, please come back to this room here and now. Thank you.

You will note that in this guided imagery session that there is no mention of anxiety. In fact, I did not know anything about that except her opening comments that she was anxious and that it had started about six months ago. Her closing affect was remarkably different than the starting one where she was obviously tense. The imagery used what she had told me about her safe haven and what she needed for healing. In general terms, she was provided access to the Holy Spirit and Jesus. I emphasize here the word "guided" in this work: I was the *guide* to her own resources and memories and ability to change. There was no need to dig into the past, but work on the present and the future as Milton Erickson and others have pointed out.

Two further comments about this session. You probably noted that in the introduction I mentioned that I had asked her permission to hold her hand at some point, and that she gave me that permission. Yet, when I reached out and mentioned holding her hand, it did not move. I acknowledged that. After the session ended she told me that at that time Jesus was holding her hand! I told her that I could not compete with Jesus! At this point I gave her a small smooth flat stone that I told her I had picked up one day in the woods near the pine forest. I gave this to her indicating that it was to be her reminder of the changes she had already made. She took the stone. I ran into her sometime later (as you do in this small village), and she thanked me for the gift of the stone. I have a collection of such smooth flat small stones to give out as kinesthetic anchors for a given session. You may wish to have such small stones or other items for the same purpose.

I mentioned at the beginning of this chapter that in recent times I have used guided imagery for psychotherapy with almost all of my clients. For psychotherapy guided imagery is, in effect, a streamlined five-step model:

1 *Information gathering*—obtain sufficient information about what is troubling your client. (I generally need to know *only* that they are anxious or depressed or overweight.)
2 *Relaxation*—Have they had any experience meditating or how do they relax? (I generally suggest just paying attention to their breathing as a good method.)
3 *Safe haven*—Do they have a place they go to in their mind that is real or imaginary where they feel safe and secure? If they tell you of one, ask for some details. (You may need to suggest several possible places such as the ocean, forests, near running water, back yard, etc.)
4 *Healing modality*—What or who do they sense will help them through their current troubles, and will help them realistically resolve these difficulties? (In my experience people choose religious figures, friends,

relatives, wise persons, and healers. Note that *they pick* who or what will bring about desired change(s) now.)

5   *Closing*—State that they will be able to remember and recall everything in this session that has been helpful to them. (In general, all they need to do is find a quiet place, pay attention to their breathing, and they will re-experience the session.) Thank them for their trust and their attention and return them to the here and now.

Consider that the above five-steps effectively incorporate the essence of a psychotherapeutic session that can fit just about any concerns a client brings to a session. That is, it is easy to adapt to various situations and clients.

6.8 Commentary

In this chapter guided imagery was discussed for two main purposes: healing and psychotherapy. Also, two transcripts were included to illustrate these two approaches. What continues to be amazing to me is how words can be used to help people both physically and mentally. Both the human mind and body are miracles. A simple reframing can bring about significant change. Also, simple *inclusivity* statements and questions such as, "I wonder what it would be like to be actively depressed" and "What would it be like to happily sad?" are amazingly effective.

I do chemistry demonstration shows for school children. One of the demonstrations is about the physical and chemical properties of dry ice (solid carbon dioxide). I always tell the students that the body responds to extreme cold the same way it does to extreme heat. I then tell them that if I did not know how to handle dry ice safely I would "burn" myself. At a recent demonstration I accidentally pressed a piece of dry ice against a finger and did burn myself. Soon afterwards a "burn" blister appeared on that finger. The blister slowly decreased in size, a red covering appeared, and then in about two weeks that disappeared and I had my normal finger back. You have probably cut a finger at some time and been amazed that when it was healed that the fingerprint returned! To my mind, then, our bodies (and minds) have a remarkable resiliency to restore themselves to health. (This is sometime called "homeostasis.") I consider this to be a miracle, and that we all are miracles. I believe that this is a wonderful way to think about ourselves and our clients.

Note

1   I make no distinction between meditation, relaxation, or hypnosis since they are all manifestations of *focused attention*. In fact, this is my working definition of hypnosis (or trance).

7 Case Study 3

Marvin, Weight Control, and the Mighty M&Ms

in its shell
cautiously tasting the world
the turtle survives

Marvin is in his fifties, never married, on disability for many years, and listed his occupation (when he worked) as a chef. He simply said that he wanted to "change my eating habits." Additional information is that his current weight was about 225 lb, and that he does not like vegetables or fruits. So, he was one of my weight control clients. I never use the words "weight loss" because what people lose they can find! Also, overweight people generally are quite knowledgeable about diets (they have tried many!), know that calories count, and are "addicted" to some "no-no" foods. Marvin could not resist standard candy-coated chocolate M&Ms. I told him that I liked to start with a discussion of the physiology of weight control.

Everybody has a basal metabolism set point. That is, the way we metabolize food is automatically regulated within certain parameters so that if you occasionally over-eat that does not change your weight, and if you occasionally under-eat that also does not change your weight. The body adjusts so that with occasional over-eating food is digested less efficiently, and vice versa. The set point is changed by the amount of calories you take in daily and the amount of daily exercise you do. You can decrease the set point by drastically reducing your caloric intake or by significantly increasing your daily exercise. There is a *synergistic effect* where the most effective way to lower the set point is to consistently decrease caloric intake *and* increase exercise. Each is discussed separately in what follows.

Everyone who is interested in weight control knows or can easily find out the caloric content of what they eat. One intriguing way of doing this is that everyone knows how to *overeat* to decrease caloric intake, e.g., by eating a head of lettuce for lunch and drinking lots of water. Start them out by getting them to commit to take in 30% less calories for the foreseeable future. (Milton Erickson liked to start a client out with the *paradoxical instruction* to return the following week exactly two pounds heavier than they are at this time. Once they do this they have learned that they do have control over their weight!) You can also give them permission to desire or lust after delectable high caloric foods, knowing that they no longer have to actually eat them. That is, they can enjoy the sights and odors in a bakery without actually eating. Many over-eaters gobble down food and do not actually taste it. So, eating smaller portions (use a smaller plate) and actually slowly chewing and tasting each bite helps. Around 1900 a method for doing this was called Fletcherizing.[1] Fletcher extolled and popularized the idea that good digestion and health was obtained by chewing each bite of food up to 100 times until it was liquefied before swallowing. Tasting rather than gobbling is healthier. Calories do count!

Returning to Marvin, he told me that he just gobbled those mighty M&Ms by the handful when he felt stressed, or just out of habit. They tasted so good when they were crunched to get at the chocolate inside, or when he let the outer covering dissolve before devouring the chocolate. So, I suggested that any time he felt the urge to gorge on M&Ms that he lay out exactly one dozen of them, and eat them one at a time as slowly as he could, savoring the outer candy coating and slowly letting each piece of chocolate melt before swallowing. This suggestion would later in the session be reinforced using hypnosis.

Increasing your exercise regimen (or starting one!) is the other half of the prescription. Covert Bailey (1931–2002) was a retired author, television personality, and lecturer on fitness and diet during the 1990s. His bestselling book, *Fit or Fat*, first published in 1978, emphasized the role of aerobic exercise and weightlifting in promoting weight-loss. Here are his top 25 fitness tips (with more comments to follow—I do not go into this amount of detail in the sessions since this list is for the reader):

1 Exercise. If exercise were a pill, it would be the most widely prescribed medicine in the world.
2 Eat a balanced diet, lower in fat, lower in sugar and higher in fiber.
3 Diets don't work. Exercise is the bottom line behavior for weight management.
4 Throw away your scales. Measuring your body fat is a better indicator of health than your weight.
5 When trying to lose fat, aim for a maximum of 2 pounds a week.
6 If spot reducing worked, people who chew gum would have skinny faces.
7 Crash dieting, over-exercising, and fasting will slow down your metabolism.
8 People don't stop exercising because they grow old, they grow old because they stop exercising.
9 It's easy to lose weight. The challenge is to keep it off. Exercise works.

10 Don't worry so much about your heart rate when you exercise. Use common sense and pace yourself so you can talk.

11 When you exercise, remind yourself, "I'm building fat-burning enzymes."

12 If you get out of breath when you exercise, you're going too fast.

13 One of the best ways to reduce stress is to exercise.

14 The older you are, the more important it is that you exercise. Exercise makes bones denser. Exercise helps maintain mobility.

15 Labels don't lie, but liars write labels.

16 Statistics are like bikinis. They only reveal half the truth.

17 Upper-body weight training will help women maintain lean body mass.

18 More muscle equals less workout time.

19 Don't say, "I don't eat red meat." Say, "I don't eat greasy meats."

20 There's no such thing as cellulite. The word was dreamed up by people with products to market to describe skin with texture that shows underlying fat on some women more than others.

21 The best aerobic exercise is the one you'll do every day.

22 The best time to exercise is when you will do it.

23 If you don't seem to be getting more fit, you may be exercising too hard.

24 If you exercise more than 45 minutes 5 days a week, you aren't doing it for the sake of fitness.

25 Beware of medically monitored diet programs. If you need a doctor, there must be something wrong.

The main items to glean from Bailey's advice are: exercise needs to be part of your daily activity; weight-bearing exercises increase bone density throughout the body; the best exercises to do are those that involve the big muscles in the legs (not upper body)—so walking, jogging, step machines, etc., are better than swimming, for example; gradually increase whatever exercises you do; and item #12, which guides you to not do an exercise so vigorously that you cannot easily converse with a companion, i.e., do not get out of breath.

Again, the best way to change your metabolic set point is to *permanently* decrease your caloric intake *and* increase your daily exercising.

At this time (or near the beginning of a session) I tell my client that almost all of the successful people I know who have permanently changed a particular habit find that it is like a transcendental transformation. That is, it is like a religious conversion when a person accepts Jesus. All of a sudden there is an internal change in the person where they know, somewhere deeply inside themselves, that from now on they will eat sensibly (to change their basal metabolism rate) or stop smoking or ... It is almost like a switch has flipped internally. Their view of themselves and their world has permanently changed.

So, after going over the physiology and pointing out how this transformation is part of the needed changes, my task is then to facilitate that occurrence.

This is where hypnosis enters as a way of providing many possibilities for changing behavior. After all, the hypnotic state is one where the client is more open to suggestions. Rather than blindly making suggestions, the client can be asked if they had successfully in the past changed a significant habit, and how did they do that? If the answer is "yes," then incorporate *their method* into the hypnosis session. If it is "no," then ask them what or who would help them makes this internal change. This could be a religious figure, a healer, a power animal, a friend or family member, a writing, a symbol, or a talisman or symbolic object of some kind (like a polished stone). This is part of the guided imagery format I frequently use for this part of the session. I would also need to know if they have a preferred way of relaxing or meditating, and a "safe haven," which is real or imaginary where they go to within their mind. For Marvin, relaxation via paying attention to breathing would work. His safe haven was going to a beach (in his mind) in the Outer Banks off the Carolina coast. Also, he told me that a healing presence would help out.

I do not record these sessions, so the following is a reconstruction of what I told Marvin.

7.1 Marvin and the Mighty M&Ms

Let's start, Marvin, with you just paying attention to your breathing. Just breathing gently and easily, in and out. This breath, and the next one. This heartbeat. Slowly, easily, naturally. And, with each inhale, chest and belly softly rising. Then, with each exhale, all of those muscles just relaxing. That's right. One breath at a time.

And, within your mind now, you can just drift off to that special beach of yours in the Outer Banks. Enjoy being there. The sand and sky, and the birds flying around. And, those small shore birds just scooting along at the edge of each wave as it rolls in. Your peaceful, calm time now. And, please feel free to change or alter any of the words I use and the way I say them, so that you get exactly what you need out of this session. This breath, and the next one. You may be watching that wave as it slowly approaches the beach, rises up, falls over, and rushes up the beach, then just settling into the sand to return back to the ocean. Continuing to breathe naturally and easily.

And, now, you notice someone approaching you. And, you recognize this person as your own special healing presence. Close enough now to reach out and touch you gently, softly, easily. And, this healing presence knows just exactly where within your body and mind there is that switch that can be moved so that from this time on you will be able to easily and comfortably and simply change your eating habits. That's right, is it not? Somewhere within you where the healing presence knows this switch lives. And, you can almost feel, can you not, these changes happening within you? I don't know exactly where this is happening or how you are sensing it. Yet, yet, now there is that internal sense, conviction, knowledge—yes—that this change has occurred. There may even be a little twitch or touch or warmth or even feeling of satiety. Yes.

The healing presence is also now transferring to you the knowledge and the determination, to everywhere within your mind and body where these changes are needed so that from now on you know, you just know that, yes, I am going to be okay. Those Mighty M&Ms which used to be so tempting are just wonderful colorful dots in your memory. You might even feel an opening sense of being free at last of any temptation to … And, yet, you know that from time to time you may actually eat an M&M or two, enjoying those old sensations, and know that they do not control you any more. Wow.

And, having helped you bring about these permanent changes in your eating habits, the healing presence gently withdraws, and moves away. It may have others to help, too, does it not? And, within your mind, you can reach out and thank it for helping you.

Continuing to breathe softly, easily, and naturally. This heartbeat, and the next …

Maybe, now, to remind you of these changes, and to let you know that they have now become an integral part of you, you can pick some small natural movement like touching an ear or your nose or bringing two fingers together to remind you that, yes, you are free of those old temptations. Practice this small natural movement from time to time. And, you are on your way to a healthier body and mind. And, you also know, do you not, that the new you will attain your new set point at the weight you wish to be at for the rest of your life, will take a reasonable amount of time. That switch has flipped, those internal decisions have been made. As simple as this breath and the next one.

And, Marvin, you do know that your mind is somewhat like a recorder so that you will be able to remember whatever has been said and you have felt in this session as you need it and when you need it. All you need to do is find a quiet place, where you will not be disturbed, breathe slowly, easily and naturally, and you will be able to recall these ideas and sensations and changes.

I want to thank you for your attention and your trust. And, whenever you are ready, you can just take a deep breath or two, blink your eyes, stretch a bit, and come back to this room, here and now. Thank you.

Commentary

I saw Marvin only once, he never called back, and so I have no idea as to how this session turned out for him. This case is presented to illustrate how I work with clients who see me about weight control, and also to present for study the way that I add a short hypnosis session at the end to consolidate what has preceded it.

Note

1 Horace Fletcher (1849–1919) was an American health food enthusiast of the Victorian era who earned the nickname "The Great Masticator," by arguing that food should be chewed about 100 times per minute before being swallowed: "Nature will castigate those who don't masticate." He made elaborate justifications for his claim.

8 Case Study 4

Carol and the Curious Cough

trees along a ridge
scratch shadows against the sky
a breeze tumbles through

Carol called me and asked if I helped people who had allergies. (She had heard from a friend that I did this.) I responded that I did, and that I used the NLP (Neurolinguistic Programming) fast allergy cure model (Andreas & Andreas, 1989, pp. 37–45). We set up an appointment and I saw her once. This unusual case began with several out-of-the-ordinary events. Carol called me before I left for the meeting (held in the annex building of a local group practice) and told me that she would be late. That was okay since it gave me time to return a call about setting up another meeting. When I got to the annex I realized that I had left my hearing aids at home when I was changing clothes. There was not time to go back and fetch them. When Carol arrived from over one-half hour away she needed to use a toilet. I have a key to the main building where there is a toilet, but apparently that key was not working! Fortunately, there is a public library nearby that was open, and so Carol went there. I had already set up the room where we were going to meet so that it would be easy to visualize a floor-to-ceiling and wall-to-wall transparent barrier that is used in the NLP procedure. When Carol returned I gave her my minimal intake form to fill out and told her that I had forgotten my hearing aids. She had forgotten hers, too, and so we agreed to talk a bit louder—something that hearing aid wearers do normally! I also asked her if it would be okay to rearrange the chairs so that we would sit close enough for me to comfortably reach out and set some anchors (by touching knuckles on her hand). Carol was okay with the seating and touching. [I am giving all of this detail here to show that this session began differently in many ways than a "normal" session. Also, note that there is a more detailed discussion of the NLP fast allergy cure in Chapter 22, case study 14.]

On Carol's intake form she indicated that she was 71, married with no children, and worked in one of the helping professions. She wrote in response to "Brief statement of concern(s), and what you want out of counseling" the following, "Relief from allergy." The following is a reconstruction from notes of the ensuing session.

RUBIN (R):   Is it okay if I take a few notes?[1]
CAROL (C):   Yes.
R: What is the allergy like, and how long has it been going on?
C: It's a cough that comes and goes, and has been going on for about one and one-half years. Right now it's been around for 6–7 weeks.
R: Do you know what you are allergic to? That is, what causes it?
C: No.
R: You know that there are all kinds of allergens like foods and pollens and dust mites and pet dander. Any of those things?
C: No.

[If I know what the allergen is (or allergens are), I then suggest that she think of a counter example (which is needed in the NLP procedure). A counter example may be some fine powder to which she does not react. At this point I am thinking (furiously) about how I might adapt the process to work in some kind of "generic" way. Also, in the preamble, I pointed out that a long time ago a Viennese doctor had a patient who came into his office and started immediately showing an allergic rhinitis style reaction. When questioned, the patient responded that she was allergic to roses. The doctor pointed out that the roses on his desk were artificial! This led to my telling Carol that there were two important things to understand about allergies. The first was that allergies are a mistake of the immune system in responding to harmless things in the environment. The second is that there is a psychological component to allergic responses. The NLP fast allergy cure is designed to correct the immune system's mistake and to remove the mind's reaction to allergens. After this discussion I asked ...]

R: Can you tell me something about the circumstances when you have the allergic response? That is, when you start coughing.
C: Yes, it generally happens when I am a bit anxious, when I have to say something important.
        [This response changed the rest of the session since Carol just told me that she does not have the coughing in response to the presence of an allergen (recall that she could not name one), but to an interpersonal interaction.]
R: Tell me a bit more about that.
C: It happens when I am struggling to say something important to a client or my husband or to others.
        [Wow! This means I have to change gears, give up the NLP fast allergy cure approach, and figure out how to have Carol respond differently in those situations.]

R: Carol, I want you to know that you are really presenting me here and now with a most *challenging* difficulty. I need a bit of time to figure out how to help you. Okay?

[Note: I emphasized the word "challenging" because that was a deliberate choice on my part to both give myself some time to decide on what to do next, and also to set up an expectation that whatever I was going to come up with would be unusual, different, interesting, and tailored to her needs.]

C: Yes.

R: [I thought for a while and then decided to use a David Cheek ideomotor finger-signaling approach to deal with her "anxiety" about saying significant things in certain circumstances.] Do you know anything about ideomotor responses such as finger signaling?

C: No.

R: Well, this all started with the Chevreul pendulum. He was a famous French pharmacist who developed this in the nineteenth century. Let me demonstrate this with the Medic Alert necklace I wear. [I then demonstrated with this device saying out loud "Yes, yes, yes." and "No, no, no." as answers to simple questions like "Is today Wednesday?" "Is it night time now?" "Is my name Rubin?" "Is this the morning?" The pendulum swings in one direction for "Yes" responses and 90 degrees opposite for "No" responses. This is due to micromuscular movements. The pendulum moves in a circular fashion in response to, "Are you not ready to answer now?" References are: Cheek (1994); Rossi & Cheek (1988); Ewin & Eimer (2006).]

C: Interesting.

R: Since it is much easier to do this with finger movements, let me tell you about that. Your right hand is on the arm of the chair now. Just let your index finger be the "Yes" one, your middle finger be the "No" one, and your thumb be the "I'm not ready to answer that now." finger. Okay?

C: Yes.

R: Since you might want to use this procedure with some of the people you see, let me just say a bit more about this before we get back to exploring its use with you. Okay?

C: Okay.

R: We assume that the responses are actually generated unconsciously by your mind. So, when the finger movements are smooth (and large) they are typically due to conscious actions. When the responses are what we may call unconscious, the finger movements are smaller and erratic. [I demonstrated these two kinds of movements.]

C: Interesting.

R: It is usually easier to do this if your eyes are closed or you are just looking off into the distance. Would it be okay to close your eyes now? [She did so.] Let's now just let your fingers answer my questions about when all of these coughing responses in certain situations started. Did this start ten years ago?

C: ["No" finger moves.]

R: Thank you. Did this start more than six years ago? [Note: Always acknowledge that you have observed a finger response.]

C: ["No" finger moved.]

R: Thank you. Did this start about five years ago?

C: ["Yes" finger moves.]

R: Thank you. Do you have any idea as to why or how this started at that time?

C: ["No" finger moves.]

R: Thank you. Although you may not know about how all of this started, there is something you can do about it. Just consider now that this is five years later, and you are five years older and with more experience. So, looking back *from the future*, from this time, with all that you have learned and know about yourself at this time, would it be okay to just give up that unhelpful coughing response?

C: [Thinking for a short time before "Yes" finger moves.]

R: Wow. Thank you. Sometimes, Carol, looking back we realize that it is okay to just give up something we have done or learned back then. It is a relief to do so, is it not?

C: [Nods.]

R: Thank you. Whatever it was that started back then was probably something useful in your behavior at that time. So, would it be okay now to just thank that part of yourself that started this for helping you at that time?

C: ["Yes" finger moves.]

R: Thank you. Just go ahead now and thank that part of you. It's okay now to open your eyes. Thank you. A while back I was at a presentation done by Kay Thompson, a dental surgeon, who was a great user of hypnosis. She was also quite adept at self-hypnosis. At that meeting she told us that she had some trouble in public speaking in choosing just the right words. So, she would use time distortion to help her. [Carol looked a bit puzzled at this comment.] What she did she told us is that she would slow time down enough so that she could think about and choose exactly what she wanted to say. Not all of us can do that, but it is interesting to know, is it not?

C: Yes.

R: You know, Carol, that I usually start out a session with a question I learned from Mary Goulding. Since you might find this question useful in your own work, it is, "What are you willing to change now?" In this regard, are there any things from your past that you would like to give up or change now? [She nodded "Yes."] Would it be okay to work on those things now?

C: Yes.

R: You know that I use hypnosis from time to time. If that is okay with you, just find a comfortable position in that chair, and close your eyes. Thank you. [Carol does this, and I proceed.] We can start with you just paying attention to your breathing. [After my usual comments on this, I went into the next stage.] Just continue to breathe softly and easily and naturally now. That's right. This breath, and the next one. Now, looking back on your life and who you are now, are there any other things in your life that you would like to just give up and forget about and move on? You can just answer with your fingers. [She raises her "Yes" finger.] Thanks. Good. You know that sometimes it is useful to have a little help in doing that, in making those changes in your life. So, just imagine now that you have near you, and with you, a powerful healer/helper who can make those changes come about easily and comfortably. I do not know who that would be, but you do, do you not? ["Yes" finger raises.] Thank you. And now, somehow, somehow, that person, that healer/helper, just smooths away the past things that had troubled you. They may just vanish into the air, or dribble out the ends of your fingers, or pass through your feet and shoes down into the earth to disappear forever. Good. And, now, thank that healer/helper for being with you at this time. And, you know that if you need such help again, sometime in the future, all you have to do is find a quiet place, pay attention to your breathing, and ask the healer/helper to be with you to easily bring about those changes. Good.

Continuing now to breath comfortable and easily. And, Carol, I want to thank you for your attention and your trust and your confidence. Challenges can sometimes be quite interesting, can they not? And at this time, you can take a deep breath or two, perhaps blink your eyes and stretch a bit, and come on back to this room here and now. Yes, and Yes, and thank you.

[Carol looked very much at peace and relaxed. I then said:] Carol, I would like to give you a little gift. You may have noticed here on the table a jar filled with small smooth stones. Please reach in and take one. That stone will serve as a reminder of everything that has happened here this evening that you would like to remember and keep with you. [She took one of the stones and thanked me. I then asked her:] Is there anything else you would like to talk about now?

C: No. I got what I came for. Thank you.

R: I also need to thank you since you really challenged me to come up with some useful things for you. This was not one of those routine sessions. It also began in a rather odd way, did it not? [She laughed.]

C: Yes it did.

[At that point I closed up the place where we were meeting and walked with her out to our cars. She seemed to be quite relaxed and had a big smile on her face.]

Commentary

There is much to comment upon on this session, which was somewhat extraordinary and different for me. It started with Carol calling and stating she would be late. I got to the meeting room early and discovered in my haste to change clothes and leave that I had left my hearing aids behind. When Carol arrived it turned out she had to use a rest room—I could not get into the main building and I had to direct her across the street to the public library, which has rest rooms. When she returned we settled down in our meeting room, the one I had set up to implement the NLP fast allergy cure. I mentioned that I had forgotten my hearing aids and asked her if she would speak a bit louder. She then told me that she had also forgotten her hearing aids! An interesting start.

My opening questions about her allergy elicited the fact that she did not know what she was allergic to, although she had a good idea as to when the coughing started. When I asked her in what circumstances she had this coughing response, her answer changed the entire session since it was not in response to an allergen but only in certain situations. So, this was not an allergy for which she needed help, but the situations. At this point I did not know what to do next, and I needed some time to think about alternative approaches that might be relevant. I also had to take into account that she was a helping professional. I do not know what inspired me at this point to look at her and simply state, "You know, you are really challenging me with this. I do not know what to do at this point, and I need some time to think about it." In *retrospect* I believe that these comments were the change points in the session. I had in effect told her (or implied) that: (1) I was taking her concerns seriously; (2) they were significant and important; (3) she was "challenging" me (which made her an unique and special client); (4) I needed some time to think about what to do; and (5) what I was going to propose was probably going to be different, and even surprising. I decided that I would use David Cheek's simple and direct method for change, i.e., I would use ideomotor finger signaling to lead her straight into a change mode. (See references for Cheek's work.)

As indicated in the session reconstruction above I illustrated the use of a Chevreul pendulum, and also ideomotor finger signaling. [Note that it easiest to use finger signaling by specifying which fingers are "No," "Yes," and "I am not ready to answer now," rather than have the client to choose the finger assignments.] This procedure was novel for Carol, and I explained more about it than usual since as another professional I thought that she might perhaps want to add this way of working with clients to her own repertoire. When working with other professionals it is not unusual for me to occasionally explain what I am doing and why. I also recall telling Carol that she could use ideomotor finger signaling for herself when she wanted to query her own body (or mind) about what was going on in her and her life. [Incidentally, I have a niece who uses the Chevreul pendulum to help her make business decisions!]

I also used the hypnosis segment via a modified *guided imagery* approach to provide Carol with a way of resolving (somehow![2]) whatever other concerns were troubling her. That is, I was aware that there might be other issues in her life and decided why not use the time we had together to also resolve for her anything else that was outstanding.

Finally, I will emphasize again the use of providing an anchor via the small polished stones I give away at the end of sessions. My clients appear to really like those stones and remembrances. [Is that like giving a child a lollipop or other candy as s/he leaves the doctor's or dentist's office?] Also, it must have been evident to Carol that I really enjoyed meeting her and the session we had together.

Notes

1   I invariably start a session with asking permission to take notes. I also generally point out that the notes are not legally confidential (as with a lawyer or medical doctor), and that there are some circumstances where I would have to show them. I also tell clients that I keep sparse notes.

2   I consider the word "somehow" to be one of the magic words used in hypnosis and psychotherapy. It gives the client the opportunity to do a transderivational search (an internal one) in which they can discover and apply images and ideas and possibilities and choices that are unique to them and their life history.

9 Rapport and the Therapeutic Alliance

firefly flashes
illuminate the night air
lightning the way to love

9.1 Introduction

At the initial therapy session two strangers meet for the first time. There are certain expectations on the part of each of these individuals. The client expects that the therapist will help him/her find ways of feeling better about themselves, about coping better with the difficult aspects of their lives, and that this will come about within some reasonable time frame. The therapist expects that his/ her therapeutic skills and training will be adequate to bring about the desired changes in the client's life, again within a reasonable amount of time. Almost all current therapy is face-to-face (f2f) and requires that both parties *listen* to each other, with the client responding to the therapist's questions, comments, and statements. That is, this is *talk* therapy in contrast with medication, physical manipulation, movement, and art therapy, for example. (By contrast my late colleague and old friend Luciano L'Abate had promulgated and written extensively about the usage of workbooks being the coming way of doing therapy and replacing f2f therapy. Workbooks lead a client through a series of steps that are skillfully constructed to guide the client to useful outcomes. These workbooks are available online, and are also implemented as *distance writing*. An excellent starting point in exploring the use of workbooks is the book edited by L'Abate (2004), its title being informative, *Using Workbooks in Mental Health. Resources in Prevention, Psychotherapy, and Rehabilitation for Clinicians and Researchers*. There is an extensive literature on workbooks and distance writing.) This chapter is concerned with f2f therapy.

So, the expectations of *both* persons matter, and *words* matter. The setting of the room matters, too, but not as much as the physical attitudes of each person, what they look like to each other, their postures, and their faces. It has been said that people make almost instant judgments of others by just looking at them. There is not much I can do about what I look like and my features and who I am. Clothes may be very important to some people and not others. Since I wear clothes for comfort and utility, I do not pay much attention to this. (When I attend conferences I note that there are many of my male colleagues who always wear jackets, if not suits. There are others who are always casually dressed. The norm when I started my teaching career in chemistry was suits or jackets and ties.) That first impression is important and needs to be inviting and genial and cordial. After that, and this happens quickly, it is words, words, words: what they are, and how they are delivered and received.

This, then, is all about building rapport with the client, making meaningful contact, and establishing an atmosphere that is conducive to working together towards the client's goals. This has also been written about as establishing a "therapeutic alliance." To this end it is important to point out the role of pacing and leading. That is, once you are in tune with, on the same frequency, standing on the same ground, in contact with, and speaking the same language you are *pacing* the client in his/her own way of existing in the world. You are *sympatico*, if you will. We all know that we are more comfortable (generally) with people of our own sex, backgrounds, ethnicity, religion, country, and family. When strangers meet they quickly work on establishing commonalities. Some ways of enhancing this follow. The advantage of pacing someone in some way or ways is that you can then *lead* them into changes. After all, clients come to us because they are stuck and they expect us to help them change.

9.2 Pacing Body (Postural) Language

We live three-dimensionally in the world in terms of our posture. We can sit directly opposite each other or position our chairs at various angles to each other. (The days of sitting behind a desk or beside or behind someone on a couch are over.) An angle of about 120 to 145 degrees appears to be optimum, and better than sitting directly opposite. A separation of one to two feet is good. The chairs should be comfortable. Some therapists who use hypnosis have a "hypnosis chair," others have a recliner. I find that two comfortable arm chairs work well, and that if I use hypnosis in a session, that the client can easily find a comfortable position. Occasionally, I will ask a client's permission to hold a hand. Then, the chairs have to be close enough to do that comfortably.

Matching how the client sits in the chair is pacing, and this needs to be done casually by adopting no more than one or two of the client's positions. That is, exact mirroring is noticed and can make the client uncomfortable. Cross your legs, ankles, arms, but not all of them! Does the client lean forward or back or tilt sideways? Is his head erect or relaxed? Does she make eye contact or not? Is their posture closed or open? *Whatever you pace and match needs to be done subtly.* Do they tap a foot or move their leg continually up and down? The idea is to pace body posturing outside of awareness.

The most important physical thing to match is the breathing pattern and rate of the client (again, subtly!). Our breathing patterns are unconscious, and pacing them connects on a visceral level. A child sitting on your lap while reading to them will automatically match your breathing and heart rates. When using hypnosis it is especially helpful if the delivery of your words matches your client's breathing patterns. This, then becomes an unconscious pacing since most of the time the client's eyes are closed or unfocused. When your client's eyes are closed (or unfocused) you can change the *locus* of your voice to emphasize certain words or phrases since they are unconsciously aware of the origins of your voice. If you slowly change your breathing pattern, the client will follow it, and this can be useful at times.

A way to practice postural pacing is to go to a mall and just follow people and match how they move or just stand around. You can almost literally walk in their footsteps!

9.3 Verbal Pacing

The way that a person speaks is characteristic of who they are. Do they speak: loudly or softly, quickly or slowly, rhythmically or straight, with a regional or ethnic or national accent, raspingly or haltingly or smoothly, agitated or calm, and dramatically or prosaically. There are many many ways of speaking, which one do you match (subtly)? Generally, you can connect with your client by pacing in only one of these ways. Remember that mimicking is to be avoided. From time to time it may be useful to use pacing to lead the client into a less agitated state or a more energetic one. Acting training can help develop these skills. Or, you can just have some fun with friends or family by practicing on them.

9.4 Representational Systems and Eye Accessing Cues

Neurolinguistic Programming (NLP) has made major contributions to the use of language in psychotherapy (Bandler & Grinder, 1975; Grinder & Bandler, 1976). One of them has to do with representational systems. We function in the world in terms of language, both externally and internally. Although there is some skepticism about this, I have found that it is useful to believe that people have a preferred way of speaking, i.e., using words that are primarily visual, auditory, or kinesthetic (body sensations). You can practice listening for this in groups or with individuals or on media. Here are a few examples of each (and some unspecified words):

- Visual: see, picture, clear, visual, focus, eye, look, view, draw, appear, show, and foggy
- Auditory: say, tone feedback, tune, sounds good, talk, hear, shout, rhythm, rings a bell, sounds like, said, and spoken
- Kinesthetic: handle, firm, force, build, grasp, reach, touch, solid, feel, hold, go around, fluid, grind, nail down, and concrete
- Unspecified: think, sense, judge, assume, allows, learn, motivate, thought, discover, agree, believe, decide, guess, use, allow, know, and understand.

If you recognize a preferred representational system in the words your clients use, then it is useful to respond to them in the same representational system. If you are not certain of the representational system of your client, then you may wish to respond in some way in all three representational systems. When I do public presentations I frequently (and consciously) use several representational systems. This is just one more idea that can be useful in establishing rapport.

The observation of eye movements can provide some cues as to the client's thinking. In NLP this is referred to as "eye accessing cues." Again, there is some question as to how well-established is this phenomenon. Simply put, there are six directions a person's eyes may move when they are talking, and it is posited that each direction indicates that the client is in a particular thinking mode or internal state. They are (the speaker's eye movement, i.e., you are looking *at* the speaker):

- Kinesthetic States: down and to the right
- Auditory Internal (auditory internal dialogue or messages): down and to the left
- Auditory Constructive (constructing sounds and words): directly to the right
- Auditory Recall (accessing remembered auditory sounds): directly to the left
- Visual Construction (constructing a mental image or picture): up and to the right
- Visual Recall (accessing stored mental images or pictures): up and to the left.

Again, this can be useful in the sense that you are aware of the client's internal thinking and states. This might lead you to asking questions like: "What are you thinking/feeling/seeing hearing now?" The responses can lead you into how you proceed in the interaction with client.

9.5 Anchors and Anchoring

NLP (and other disciplines) has developed an useful concept called "anchoring," which is the obtaining of a *conditioned response* by an associated stimulus. This has also been called "operant conditioning" in the field of behavioral modification (also Pavlovian and Skinnerian conditioning). That is, we can consider *anchoring to be any stimulus that elicits a consistent response*. The hand-shaking response is one of these: someone raises their right hand and you automatically raise your own hand. Thus, in one sense, you cannot *not* anchor in interaction with another person. There are many ways to "set" anchors: touch, sound of voice, hand movements, cue words, odors, tastes, body postures, voice location, physical surroundings, and other stimuli. The sense of smell is connected to a primitive part of the brain, and is perhaps the most powerful of stimuli. If I suggested that you now think about a time when you were young and your mother was baking something special and ask you to inhale deeply through your nose, you will almost instantly go back to some childhood time (a "regression") and re-experience being in a kitchen (or nearby) enjoying and experiencing that entrancing odor. How can anchoring be used in a therapeutic setting?

Of the various types of anchoring mentioned above the one that is easiest to use and also has what may be described as a *kinesthetic over-ride* is touch. There are two NLP procedures that I have used with clients that involve touch, and they are the "fast allergy cure," and the "fast phobia cure." In both of these anchoring special states by touching different knuckles or places on a shoulder, for example, are used. I am not going to describe those procedures here: if you are interested, you can just search the Internet for those terms and you will find the details as to how to do them.[1] (It does take some skill and practice to do them effectively, however.) Remember, permission must be obtained before touching a client. Kinesthetic anchors need to be placed exactly so you can accurately reproduce the anchor. Knuckles are good for this. The amount of pressure used in a physical touch anchor can be used to indicate the intensity of that anchor. One of the simplest anchors you can use in your office (assuming you have several chairs in it), is a "guided imagery" or "hypnosis" chair.

9.6 Anchoring and Remen's Healing Circle

Remen's preparation for surgery healing circle uses a small smooth stone as an anchor (see section 3.2B). I have a jar of small smooth polished stones of various sizes and shapes and colors. At the end of a session (involving hypnosis or not), I may give my client a stone from this collection, or let them pick one. This "physical" and solid anchor is to remind them of what has gone on in the session that they wish to recall. Another anchor that I have the client rehearse has to do with them practicing a given behavior or recalling a particular state when it is needed in the future by choosing some simple movement or action that is natural. This may be something like holding two fingers together, clasping their hands, making a loose fist, touching their hair or an ear or nose or chin. An example of this is a client who has difficulty doing public presentations. I have them rehearse in their mind what they have learned about how to be comfortable and at ease in such a situation, and to *anchor* those feelings of comfort and ease with the natural motion we have rehearsed. One anchor might be for them to touch the stone that anchors their desired state in a pocket and just contact it before whatever the event is for which they have prepared. (They might put the stone on the lectern, for example.) These are some ways of anchoring changed behavior(s) for an individual client.

I have adapted Remen's healing circle in several ways that can be used in group settings.

In a psychotherapy group where one of the clients is stuck this person can pick a stone out of the bowl and ask the group for guidance and help. Then the stone is passed around the group with each person in turn telling a brief story about a time in their life when they were having a particular difficult time coping and what it was they got them through that time. They each end with, "I put in this stone for you love/courage/internal strength/a wonderful memory/a special idea that someone gave me/encouragement/a sense of belonging/God's love/wisdom for you." The stone is then given to the requester to keep. At this point the leader of the group might ask everyone to hold hands while s/he does a healing meditation based on the spoken themes. The requester may or may not tell the group what it is that is troubling him or her, i.e., they wish to keep this as a personal secret that the group honors.

There are many groups focused on particular issues like: cessation of smoking, weight control for overweight people (I do not use the phrase "weight loss" since if someone loses something they can find it!), alcoholism, addiction to drugs (I do not use the phrase "substance abuse" since it is not the substance that is abusing), wife or husband or child abuse, sexual molestation, rapists, depression, anxiety, anorexia or bulimia, sleep disorders like insomnia and sleep apnea and narcolepsy, obsessive compulsiveness, etc., in each of these kinds of support groups (including those devoted to particular physical diseases). In each of these kinds of groups an individual member can receive support and coping strategies and ideas via the procedure described in the previous paragraph. The person focused on gets both a *physical anchor*, a sense that they are not alone with this concern or trouble, and ways of working their way out of it.

The first variant I used was one of dealing with grief. I did this initially in a group of about 40 people, and later in a group that may have been as large as 200. I explained the process to the group and asked for four to six volunteers who were willing to talk about a time in their life when they were grieving, and what it was that go them through that time. They each picked a stone out of the bowl, and, holding it up, they briefly told their story and put into their stone what helped them. I then had them put their stones back in the bowl, stirred the stones, and they then each picked up another stone. I then had everyone hold hands up in front with the stone in their left hand and we held hands with people in the audience who held hands with each other. The healing meditation I delivered was about all of the stones in the bowl having been imbued with all of the various ways the volunteers put into their stones, and that somehow via us all holding hands those characteristics would now be available to everyone in the room. At the end audience members who had a particular need for this were invited to go to the bowl and take away a stone for themselves. This procedure can be adapted to any of the concerns and groups mentioned above.

9.7 Some Closing Comments

This chapter has described a bunch of methods and ideas about achieving rapport with single clients and also with groups. Therapy happens when the client and the therapist are functioning in the world in parallel and connected ways. As therapists, then, we are both guides and companions in finding new ways to function and live. This may be described by one of my mother's favorite sayings, "One hand washes the other." So be it …

Note

1 Both of these procedures are described later as case studies with transcripts and commentary and guidelines. See Chapter 22 for the fast allergy cure case study and Chapter 23 for the fast phobia cure case study.

10 Case Studies 5 and 6

Sammy and Self-Regard and Normalizing Norman

parent, adult, child
contaminate each other
bringing scripts to life

10.1 Introducing Sammy and Norman

Sammy found me through the Milton H. Erickson Foundation when he asked for someone in Ohio who used Ericksonian hypnosis and psychotherapy.[1] Sammy lives in Northern Ohio and is perhaps the client I have seen more than any other, although this is best described as *sequential single-session therapy* (sessions in 2008, 2012, 2014, 2017, and 2018). His friend Norman also saw me sequentially: 7/2012, 6/2013, 8/2014, 8/2015, 9/2018, and 4/2019. In between sessions I have occasionally heard from Norman, and much more frequently from Sammy via email exchanges.

In his first session with me Sammy wrote the following two sentences in terms of what he wanted out of counseling: "To realize my full potential" and "I want to grow up and act like a mature adult." (He was 32 at the time.) Hypnosis was used along with Narrative Therapy in terms of "exorcizing" his demons. His next session was three years later and he stated he was stuck at 36 years of age and wanted a sense of direction in his life. After some time with the Miracle Question this was integrated into a hypnosis session. Sammy left with more hope. Two years later he had finished a program to become a physical therapist, had met a young lady, and seemed to be moving along in a positive way. I used some of Steve Andreas's negative self-talk approaches and hypnosis (see sections 12.4 and 12.5). Sammy returned for another session after three more years in which I used a "helper" in a hypnosis session to help him with decision making. He also picked a smooth stone as an anchor for the session. We ended with a brief intervention to help him with weight control. His last session was about one year later. By then he had married and lost his job and found another one. In this session (some of which will be presented in the following case study) we apparently got around to some fundamental difficulties in his life. Since it turned out that there were several "witch" messages from his father (deceased five years before) the Gestalt Therapy two-chair approach was used to resolve long-standing "witch" messages from his father. This was followed by an Erickson "February Man"[2] hypnosis session to fill in for his dad and to provide valid-ation and recognition. The session ended with a Narrative Therapy exorcism of a controlling internal ogre that was still haunting and controlling him. An email from Sammy a few months later indicated that he had lost another job. I suggested that he do a Gestalt Therapy two-chair session by himself to resolve whatever was disturbing him at this time (in lieu of visiting me for a session). This is where things stood until the 4/2019 session whose summary follows after my reconstruction of the one on 9/2018.

10.2 Case Study 5: Sammy and Self-Regard (9/2018)

Somehow Sammy manages to do "self-sabotage" (his words) in his employment. He is quite sociable and outgoing and has worked as a salesman from time to time where his personality helped until he "somehow" lost the job or interest in it. He has a lot of energy and exudes confidence, yet there is an underlying lack of self-regard and surety that belies the outward confidence. So, for the first time in this session he talked about his father and the fact that his father did not recognize his achievements or show love. This non-recognition appeared to be the central issue in his life, and suggested to me that what was now needed was a Gestalt Therapy two-chair experience. (His father had died five years before, which removed the opportunity to directly meet with him and work this through.)

Sammy started talking to his father who was in the chair opposite him. At appropriate times I asked Sammy to switch chairs and be his father responding to whatever Sammy said. This exchange went back and forth about seven times until a resolution was reached in which (acting as his father with remembered voice quality and mannerisms) his father told him he loved him and secretly(!) admired his accomplishments (he could not bring himself to do this—prior to this time—overtly). In the exchange they both exhibited much emotion. We had a discussion about what had just happened, and this time was used to slow Sammy down and to get him to be quieter. [Frequently, after one of these sessions the client needs time to incorporate what has gone on and to (in a way) save it so that it becomes part of their history.]

At this point I felt that more was needed to solidly embed in Sammy what had just happened. [I recalled Erickson's use of being the "February Man" with a woman who was concerned about her pregnancy and becoming a mother. Erickson provided the knowledge and guidance that she needed to be a mother.] Fortuitously, this session with Sammy actually occurred in February! I became his father for the (reconstructed) hypnosis session that follows.

10.3 February Man Script for Sammy

Sammy, I just told you the story about Milton Erickson and how being in the identity of a "February Man" he helped this young woman. I am now going to be your dad in this month of February. If you are comfortable closing your eyes now, please do so. And, be sure that you are in a comfortable position. Continuing to breathe softly and easily. Naturally. This breath and the next one. This heart beat and ... That's right. Chest and belly softly rising with each inhale. And, then with each exhale, all of those muscles just relaxing. This breath and the next one.

I don't know exactly where we are going to meet. You will know. And just imagine now that you and I—me as your father and you now at an earlier age, or now—are together. I have some things to tell you that I could not do back then. As you know, I have had a hard life and my parents were not the best. So, I found it really difficult to talk to you and to tell you anything good. I thought you needed to grow up tough like I did. Okay? You did, and you became your own person. How could I tell you that I loved you and that I was proud of the things that you accomplished? I could not then. So, here we are in February, a cold time. I hope you are listening as I (through Rubin) are telling you things that I want you to know. It may be difficult to believe after all of this time. Listen. Please listen. You were a good son. I was proud of you even though I never told you. And, although you may not believe this, there are a few of my friends who could confirm that. Okay?

So, here you are, all grown up and married and working. From way back then—and now—believe me son when I say that I was proud of you, I believed you would become something in your life, and I loved you. Yes, I loved you in my own way.

And, now I must leave. And I leave you with my blessing and my words. Farewell, and fare well.

Sammy, it is time for you to think and ponder and believe and go deep within yourself. Continuing to breathe slowly and deeply and easily. Just one breath at a time, as life is just one breath at a time. And, perhaps, within your mind, you will be able to thank your father and the February Man for this visit and what they have shared with you. Know that you will be able to recall what you heard today when and as you need it.

So, now, just taking a deep breath, blinking your eyes, return to this room here and now. Thank you.

[Sammy appeared to be deeply moved by this experience, and said nothing for a while. When he started to talk again he told me that he needed some additional help at this time to be able to deal with what he called his internal controlling ogre. I then suggested that we do some more work, and that it be to exorcize that ogre. He agreed. The next section is about the Narrative Therapy[3] related work we did to wind up this session.]

Exorcizing an Ogre: After explaining that we are sometimes controlled in our behavior by some kind of evil spirit within us, I ask the client about this idea and they almost always agree. I then ask if they would give this evil spirit a name or symbol. This provides background information on which to build the rest of the session. Finally, the client is asked if they can think of some effective way of getting rid of O. I use *their way* or create a reasonable one (as I did with Sammy).

A Exorcism Part of Session

Just get comfortable now, and let your eyes gently close. Sammy, we can use your imagination and a bit of help from one of your helping spirits, can we not? Breathing softly and easily and naturally. O has been giving you trouble for quite a while hasn't he? [I decided to make O male.] And, yet you have been able to resist O from time to time and put him in his place and ignore him. You and I know that despite O you have been able to take care of yourself, get a degree, work well in your new profession, and find a wonderful woman to marry you. All I can say to that is "Wow!" And now it is time to get rid of O completely.

Just imagine and feel now that what you have been able to accomplish in your life is the dominant and the strong inner part of you. At the same time, you also have with you the knowledge that your father did love you, and in his own way recognized your accomplishments. I don't know where within your body O lives, yet you do. And, now, something interesting and powerful is going to happen. Somehow, somehow, your inner strength and abilities are marshaling themselves and slowly and inexorably moving O from your body and mind. Easily and simply exuding O so that he is outside now and moving away. There is a sudden lightness inside you now, is there not, as O is pushed solidly and powerfully up and away and rises higher and higher into the sky. O is now soaring out of the earth's orbit and accelerating towards the sun at light speed. And, in a few minutes O has burned to a crisp in the sun's heat, disappearing forever from your life. Breathing softly and easily and naturally. What a relief. And you know, do you not, that you are free at last. Free at last to be who you are and who you were meant to be.

You know, Sammy, that from now on O is gone forever and completely. And, you are now you, ready to move on and just simply be. There may be a time when you need to recall part of this again. At that time, find a quiet place where you will not be disturbed, close your eyes, breathe easily and you will recall all what you have accomplished here today. I want to thank you, Sammy, for your trust and confidence and attention. And, when you are ready, take a deep breath or two, stretch a bit, blink your eyes, and come back to this room here and now. Thank you. This kind of "exorcism" or way of removing a controlling part of someone must appear strange to many of you. Yet, I have used this procedure in a variety of ways with many clients and have never had one who did not accept these ideas and participate in this experience. A "mantra" in Narrative Therapy is that, "The client is not the problem, the problem is the problem." This removes from them the onus of being bad or no good or evil or helpless. There is this other "thing" within them that is responsible for their misery and difficulties and limitations. When this "thing" has been neutralized and removed and made to disappear, then they can be "themselves" and free of this insidious control. (I must admit that I have been amazed from time to time that this procedure works!)

[A final note involves an email from Sammy in which he told me that he was fired from his current job and did not know why. I suggested in a return email that he now knew how to do the two-chair exercise and that he would be able to work his way out of this current difficulty by confronting the part of himself that had led to this. As I have not had a response, I am assuming that he was able to do this.]

4/20/19 Session: Sammy is now working at a different job, and one that he likes and gives him many opportunities. He has some new goals in his life. The relationship with his wife is excellent. (He continues to be overweight, though.) He has been practicing Buddhism and is quite knowledgeable about this. Before doing a guided imagery session, I posed a David Cheek ideomotor finger signaling question. (Cheek uses this kind of signaling to find out when the particular difficulty started, and then goes back to that time and asks the indicated question.) "Now that you are older and know when and how this started (a teacher telling him when he was quite young that he would mess things up in his life), is it okay now to give up that response and realize that you are a different and competent person now?" He responded "Yes." I then suggested that he write out this early "witch" message and then permanently get rid of it some way like burning it or burying it or throwing out in the trash. Sammy agreed to do this.

The three things I needed information about for the guided imagery session were: (1) method of relaxing or meditating—he pays attention to his breathing; (2) the safe haven was his extra bedroom in his house, which is his relaxation and meditation space; and (3) what is the healing modality that will guide and help him through his current difficulties? This latter part was related to his Buddhist practice and was a kind of universal connectedness to the universe and otherness. I introduced for this the idea of the "oceanic experience." [One definition of this is,

> The experience, usually brief and completely unexpected, of being at one with the entire universe, and of feeling a deep meaning and purpose to every part of existence. It is often accompanied by feelings of compassion and love for all beings.

Another, related to Sigmund Freud is,

> In a 1927 letter to Sigmund Freud, Romain Rolland coined the phrase "oceanic feeling" to refer to the sensation of being one with the universe. According to Rolland, this feeling is the source of all the religious energy that permeates in various religious systems, and one may justifiably call one-self religious on the basis of this oceanic feeling alone, even if one renounces every belief and every illusion.

This seemed to be what Sammy was describing.]

These three items were incorporated into a guided imagery session that naturally involved Sammy going into a trance state. I am only going to recon-struct here one part of the hypnosis session since it is something that I have used from time to time with clients. This is a way of connecting with the client without making physical contact, and also was very much a part of Sammy's Buddhist practice.

10.4 Script for Sammy's Oceanic Buddhist Experience

[When talking about the oceanic experience and connecting with that uni-versality I said something like what follows.] As you listen to me now you are aware that my voice is carried through the air in sound waves that connect with your ears, and these vibrations enter your body and are dispersed through it. So, these very vibrations are a way of our sharing this time and space. Also, we are both breathing in the same air space now. There are those who believe that we may even be breathing in at this time a few molecules of air that were breathed in by people who lived millennia ago, and the molecules got dispersed by winds throughout our atmosphere. It might even be that somehow a few of these molecules have come from India and might actually have been breathed by the Buddha himself. What an interesting idea to be sharing air with all those who came before us, and even all animals and plants. Continuing to breath softly and easily. So, the very air we are breathing now is here to help you at this time of your life to guide you and be with you when you need their healing presence. Softly and easily. And, you will be able to recall these ideas and feelings and presence whenever you need them. They will be there with you in your meditating and peaceful room.

I have not reconstructed here the entire hypnosis session with Sammy, and only indicate that he appeared to get out of it what he wanted in terms of his needs at this time. The image of connecting via sound vibrations is one I have used a number of times. In conclusion, I expect that Sammy will contact me again sometime in the future to continue these "sequential single-session" therapy visits.

Notes

1 I believe I am the only one on their referral list in Ohio and Indiana and other nearby areas. Although Ericksonian work is quite popular worldwide (many Affiliated Institutes) for some reason hypnosis is not as popular in the United States.
2 See *The February Man: Evolving Consciousness and Identity in Hypnotherapy* (Erickson & Rossi, 1989).
3 See White and Epston (1990), Epston and White (1992), Freedman and Combs (1996), and White (2007).

11 Case Study 6

Normalizing Norman

what is my essence?
the simple man asked of me
and I answered "yes"

When I first met Norman he was 20 years old. I saw him five times (2012–2018). His opening concern was that he puts a lot of pressure on himself, and then he added that he had nothing to talk about. He has low activation energy in terms of working on school demands and also in general. We chatted for a while and he mentioned that he had practiced yoga and meditation. We had a short hypnosis session. My impression was that just being able to share his concerns with an older person who listened to him and took him seriously was what he needed at that time.

He returned about one year later and reported that his relationships with people were now more useful and productive. He's on the dean's list at school and working part-time. There was lots of chatting. I introduced him to Viktor Frankl's work and philosophy, especially in Frankl's terms of man's search for meaning. In the hypnosis session (he is a good subject) the imagery was illuminating light and energizing. At the end of the session I gave him a set of worry stone beads to "protect" him from noxious people. [You will note that I like to give clients concrete anchors for what goes on in sessions.]

One year later, Norman returned. My sense was that he just liked being able to chat openly with an older person, and that this stabilized and energized him somehow. [I noted that his grandfather had died, and that his mother has significant dementia.] We did several as-if things, chatted quite a bit, and ended with a hypnosis session to consolidate what had gone on in the session. He had also read Frankl and done many personal reframings.

Norman returned in three years with his girlfriend (Judy) who wanted the session as a birthday gift to him. He had finished college, said he was stressed at times, and also had much anxiety before going to sleep. I suggested the guided imagery approach and he settled on these three items: (1) relaxation via counting breaths and breathing; (2) his safe haven was lying on a couch near a window with sunlight coming through; and (3) that the healing entity he preferred was a healing light. All of this was built into the guided imagery session. I felt that a bit more was needed so I guided both Norman and Judy through the Miracle Question approach. Judy followed the procedure silently while Norman responded directly as I guided him through his day post-miracle. They both took one of my polished stones as anchors for the session, and I sent them copies of my sleep and relaxation CD and the guided imagery CD. Following the session they sent me a card stating, "We both thought we would send this 'happy' card as a way to say thank you. We are already seeing changes and enjoying the results of our visit. Thank you for all that you do." [I must say that I rarely receive feedback from my clients.]

Commentary

The title of this case study uses the work "normalizing." This is one of the things that we do as therapists since clients frequently come to us with a sense of being different from the other people in their lives. They even feel a bit unusual, too. So, we reframe these self-images and feelings to be "normal" in the sense that this is just a part of living and growing up and experiencing life. There is a sense of relief in clients to know that other people have gone and are going through the same questioning of their lives.

In the Charlie Brown support group I facilitated normalizing is generally one of the things that new members need. They may have joined the group because they have been recently diagnosed with a life-challenging disease like cancer. In their opening remarks they (almost tentatively) tell us that they are depressed and have been depressed. These remarks seem to imply that there is something wrong with being depressed. At this point I generally say nothing and other members of the group spontaneously share their experiences of being depressed when first diagnosed, and that they go through depressed states periodically. They tell the new member that this has been "normal" for them. In essence they are saying that it is certainly okay to be depressed from time to time. This is just as normal as experiencing hope, and just living as usual while all of this medical "stuff" goes on around them. No surprises at being depressed. All of this is something I reinforce with a few comments like: "I believe that everyone who has been in this support group has talked at one time or another about being depressed," and "You know, this also happens with people who do not have cancer, and just from everyday life." Sometimes these statements are received with surprise and incredulity. They are mostly received with an obvious sense of relief.

There is a classic normalizing reframe that is useful for new clients. And that is, "You know that just coming to see me (or any other therapist) takes a certain amount of courage and strength." This is a truism that acknow-ledges the doubts that frequently accompany the decision to see a therapist. Somehow, they have reached the point in their life where they are taking charge and doing something difficult, but also proactively just being alive. Why not congratulate them about this?

Since I give myself permission in my sessions with clients and in my workshops to just follow wherever my mind leads me, I find now that my mind has drifted back to the YAVIS syndrome (if you please) that I learned about in my counseling courses. The relevant class discussion was about how the different characteristics of clients affect therapeutic outcomes. That is, what are the characteristics that favor good outcomes in clients that influence the therapist to do his or her best? We were told that YAVIS clients generally had better outcomes than non-YAVIS clients. Since I forgot the origin and exact meaning of YAVIS, I simply consulted Wikipedia and reproduce their description here:

> YAVIS (sometimes "YAVIS Syndrome") is an acronym that stands for "Young, Attractive, Verbal, Intelligent, and Successful." The term was coined by University of Minnesota professor William Schofield in his 1964 book *Psychotherapy: The Purchase of Friendship* in which he claimed to have demonstrated that mental health professionals often have a positive bias towards clients exhibiting these traits. In other words, individuals with these characteristics are assumed to represent a psychotherapist's "ideal patient." Schofield explained that such a bias may in turn predispose the professional to work harder to help these clients. Such an inclination, although mostly unconscious, was thought to be driven by an expectation that clients with such traits would be motivated to work harder in therapy, thereby increasing the therapist's hope that the treatment would be effective. Further, this process would work to enhance the therapist's experience of him/herself as competent, which may help explain why YAVIS clients are unconsciously seen as more desirable.

This makes a lot of sense, and it also raises the question of what would be the opposite characteristics of a client that preclude poor outcomes? Would they be something like: **Old, Unattractive, Nonverbal, Stupid, and Unsuccessful (OUNSU)**? [This presents much for us to think about, yes?]

12 Healing Language

      it is just enough
      to hold a little girl's hand
      for a quiet walk

12.1 Introduction

When I was a boy growing up in the Bronx it was not unusual there (or elsewhere) for us to insult each other with as creative insults as we could think up. The standard reply was invariably, "Sticks and stones can hurt your bones, but words will never harm you." We all believed that incantation, even though inside we felt miserable about the insults. It was fantasy on the part of the insulter that the words would have an effect, and fantasy on our part that it would not. These insults and negative comments and words and observations used by significant people in our lives have and had long-lasting effects. As adults we can all recall the many negative things said about us by casual and power figures like our parents, siblings, "friends," and teachers: "You'll never succeed." "Who would marry you?" "Who could love you?" "You're ugly/dumb/stupid/a bum/ignorant/impossible/a brat/selfish/ isolated/always wrong/can't sing anything/can't draw/a throwback/inept/not a member of this family, etc., etc." Even though later in life we married, had children, loved and were loved, succeeded in chosen careers, etc., those negative or "witch" messages hovered in our unconscious, and even had continuing effects on how we lived and behaved and felt and thought of ourselves. WORDS CAN HARM US.

Since almost all therapists function in the f2f (face-to-face) mode via words, we need to be aware of our unconscious negative messages and sensitive to those of our clients. Steve Andreas (2012, 2014) has written two wonderful and useful books about transforming negative self-talk. They are full of practical and effective exercises, and I will use a section of this chapter to present a sampling of them. Most of the exercises are based one way or another on NLP, and most of them can simply be thought of as applications of common sense. The idea is to *reframe* and *de-potentiate* the negative self-talk which we incorporated early in our lives. ("Now that you are older, isn't it time to give up those old ideas?")

Let me cite here a really harmful message reported to me by a friend who had consulted a doctor for an evaluation of lumps in her breast. She had not heard the test results from him for a while, and she called him. He called back and she told me that this was the full message he gave her before he hung up, "You have breast cancer, and it will probably kill you." This phone call occurred over 30 years ago and presumably that doctor is no longer practicing. You should know that I talked with this friend recently, and she is still alive and active even though in the intervening time she has had some serious diseases. I believe this was a rare occurrence even decades ago, yet it is an example of the kind of thoughtless harmful messages that can occur. I wrote an entire book about healing language (Battino, 2010), and I am going to use that as a resource for the rest of this chapter (along with Andreas's contributions). There are 68 "scenarios" in my book that consist of a given situation, and examples of healing and harmful language concerning that situation (a few are presented in section 12.5).

12.2 Reprise on Useful Definitions

I have found it useful to make a distinction between the words " disease" and "illness." A *disease* is the physical manifestation of something being wrong or abnormal in the body. Diseases are things like cancer, a broken bone, pneumonia, diabetes, an abscessed tooth, prostatitis, or congestive heart failure. A normal and healthy person is free of diseases, and doctors have an enormous number of methods for curing diseases by medications, surgery, and diet change, for example. There are well-known methods for treating diabetes. (A major difficulty with treating diabetes, and other diseases, is patient compliance with medical recommendations. Some of the recommended regimens are misunderstood, some are difficult to follow, and many are just ignored.)

An *illness* is how you *feel and think* about the disease. What is the *meaning* that you give to the disease? That is, this is not the physical dimension, but the mental dimension. And, this is basically controlled by your upbringing, your family and how they think about being sick, your religion and your culture, and your own belief system. There are two questions that can be used to elicit this information: "Why do you think that you have this particular disease?" and "What does it *mean* to you?" How you respond to a diagnosis of a life-challenging disease (indeed, any disease) is controlled by and linked to how you respond to those queries. Illnesses can be healed by altering the feelings and beliefs about the disease. There are many ways to do this like reframing, accurate information, being in a support group, writing, and sharing feelings with supportive people like family or friends or therapists or ministers. In my experience, sharing *confidentially* in the support group I facilitated (Charlie

Brown) heals our members. (The word "confidential" is important here.) I have found that people will share thoughts and feelings in the support group that they feel uncomfortable sharing with family or significant others. Consider that in Native American traditions (as well as others) being healed means being back in *harmony* with Nature. Healing then means being *whole* again, and being restored to a harmonious sense of self. A significant amount of dissociation occurs with a diagnosis of a life-challenging disease. There is an unreality and strangeness at suddenly becoming someone and something else. Who is this new person? Healing, however attained, restores us to our sense of who we are. It is also not surprising in my experience that healing is often accompanied by a significant amount of curing and improvement in physical health.

To summarize, diseases are cured and illnesses are healed. For me, these distinctions are useful both linguistically and practically.

People tend to avoid the giving of what they feel is "false hope." Perhaps they feel that they are being kind to a person who has essentially just been given a death sentence, and that it is better just to accept that and tie up the loose ends of their life and "enjoy" what is left. That is, "be realistic." They are missing two things here: the first is that *we are alive* until our last breath, and that hope is a potent word in terms of marshaling healing and curing resources. Yet, it is good to be realistic. There are lots of practical things to do. At the same time, there is an important distinction between a diagnosis and a prognosis. A diagnosis is based on tests of experimentally determined statistical reliability. So, diagnoses all have "error bars" associated with them. It is important to know the magnitude of those error bars. There is a difference of "this test has a reliability of 90%" and "this other one has a reliability of 50%." A medical doctor making a prognosis is making his/her statement based on experience, which is based on the reliability of those tests! So, you may have to believe the diagnosis, but you do not have to believe the prognosis. This is why in serious cases it is vitally important to obtain second and even third opinions. (There is a remarkable book by S. S. Schneider (2005) entitled *The Patient from Hell. How I Worked with My Doctors to Get the Best of Modern Medicine and HOW YOU CAN TOO.* The title tells it all!)

I have heard Bernie Siegel state on a number of occasions, "What is wrong with hope?" With hope you go out and get more information about your disease, you get second opinions, you change your life style, and you marshal your own immune system and body and mind's healing capacities to work at full strength. It is well known that active and involved patients have better outcomes than inactive and depressed ones. Are your treatments being done "to you" or "with you?" Are you assertive and have an advocate or are you passive and rely only on "professionals?" Do you automatically and consistently request copies of all relevant documents and tests and reports, or do you assume that "they" know what they are doing and give them your blind trust? (All of my and my wife's medical practitioners know that we want these reports, and they give them to us. They even mail them when they are not available at sign-out.) Almost all health services now have websites that you can access and in which you can retrieve test results and reports. You can also bring along with you to appointments small recording devices so you can record whatever happens. Ask for permission first—I have never been refused such a request, although it was apparent this permission was occasionally given reluctantly. "Hope" sometimes needs some help.

12.3 Reframing

The way that you frame an art object, painting, or photograph, has a significant impact on how you view it. In a similar way, how buildings are sited, landscaped, and their facades created convey important information. How you "frame" yourself in clothing for different occasions can be impactful. In the previous examples you need to know your audience. The entrance to some medical facilities can be cold and scary, and to others can be warm and inviting. In interacting with people what you say and how you say it is primary if you want your communication to be healing. There are ways to linguistically reframe what you say to enhance healing.

Since you want to change how a person feels using words to enhance healing it is important to know a bit about change in psychotherapy. The book by Watzlawick et al. (1974), makes an useful distinction between first- and second-order change. A *first-order change* occurs within the system, and is generally characterized by doing more of the same. That is, if cutting taxes does not work, then cut them more. Or, if this punishment of junior does not work, then increase the punishment. With respect to the "war" on drugs, if increasing the penalties has not worked to stop the flow of drugs, then increase the punishments and criminal sentences. This occasionally works, but the advice of, "If it isn't broke, don't fix it; and if it hasn't worked, do something different," makes more sense.

On the other hand, a *second-order change* is *meta* to or outside of the system. Second-order change tactics can be characterized as being: strange, off-the-wall, paradoxical, and odd. They are essentially *not doing* more of the same. For example, European countries treat the use of "illegal" drugs as a medical problem rather than a criminal one, and have significantly smaller drug problems.

In terms of healing language, reframing works as a second-order change. The self-descriptive "inclusivity" approach is a reframe. Here are a few examples:

- What would it be like to be happily sad or energetically depressed?
- Wouldn't it be interesting to be healthily ill or energetically resting?

- What about being comfortably in easy pain or at a comfortable distance and dissociated from your pains?
- What would it be like for that pain to just be simply bothering you?
- What if that discomfort were over there and not over here?

Reframes come in two versions: content and context. Consider that no behavior in and of itself is useful or not useful. That is, every behavior will be useful somewhere, and identifying *where* is *context* reframing. Also, since no behavior means anything of and in itself, you can effectively make it mean anything: that's *content* or *meaning* reframing. The classic reframe is, "You know, it takes a great deal of courage and strength to visit a therapist for the first time." Another one is, "Coming to this support group shows that you are dedicated to helping yourself and finding out more about how to live at this time." In my early days in the Charlie Brown support group, Tom who was there to support his wife who had cancer, would say, "I come here to learn how to live a day at a time. Sometimes it is an hour at a time, and sometimes it is a minute." (Incidentally, his wife, Carolyn, graduated from a hospice program, stopped treatments even though her oncologist continued to recommend them, and lived for another 17 years.) Living one day/hour/minute at a time is a way of reframing your life. A context reframe may have the person experiment with having their troubling symptom(s) in different locations and times. With a couple presenting sexual concerns, one might suggest, "I wonder what it would be like when you start sleeping on each other's side of the bed." Also, "I wonder what would happen to your insomnia if you had your head at the foot of your bed tonight."

Here are a few gems from the collected works of Kay Thompson (Kane & Olness, 2004), a dental surgeon who was a superb hypnotist:

- It's not fair for you to let something that happened a long time ago in a different circumstance and in a different situation influence the response that you are going to have today or tomorrow. *It's not fair!* (p. 307).
- And so when you know that you know everything you need to know, even though some of it you didn't really need to know you knew, but now that you know that you don't really need to know whether you knew it, you can let yourself know everything that you need to know in order to do this, any time you know you need it (p. 156).
- It's nice to know that you can remember to forget what wasn't important to remember any way, the way you know how to do that, either by forgetting to remember it, or instead by remembering to forget it, or alternatively, perhaps you'll decide somewhere inside to remember to forget to remember or to forget to remember to forget. Either way is fine, just let your mind do the work. I know you won't mind letting your mind do that. The mind knows by itself how to mind, that's right (p. 529—wonderful confusion technique).

- [Two statements about pain.] Pain is a danger or warning signal, period. When everything that can be done and should be done, has been done, there is no longer any reason to have pain (p. 267). You can be as miserable as you need to be, but you don't have to be painful about it (p. 289).

The preceding quotations are reframes.

12.4 Transforming Negative Self-Talk

Steve Andreas has published two books on negative self-talk (2012, 2014), which contain many useful and practical suggestions about how to do this. He was an NLP practitioner and trainer, and it helps to have a bit of a background in that way of working. First, a bit of background in this section.

The (now) old approach called "Transactional Analysis" (Berne, 1964) was concerned in part with dealing with what they called "Witch Messages." They generally occurred when we were young, and were negative messages given to us by significant people in our lives: e.g., parents, siblings, friends, relatives, teachers. Often the messages were repeated frequently, especially when we misbehaved! Due to a peculiarity of the human mind many of these messages got permanently lodged there, and in effect haunted us and controlled our behavior and responses as we grew older. I know that in my own case there were messages about behavior that I grew out of in the sense that my actual accomplishments and behavior transcended the messages, but continued to exist in their miserable way even though there was "evidence" to the contrary! I still recall being startled by a comment I overheard a chemistry colleague say about me early in my career that he wished he was as calm and as good as I was. That is, I did not seem to be troubled by the doubts he had about himself (and which I continued to secretly have …). This overheard comment did have a positive effect on how I thought about myself, though. To generalize what happened to me suggests that when other more powerful magicians or wizards or mature wise men and women overtly recognize positive characteristics and behaviors *they* can countermand and even eradicate the original witch message(s). Also, experience can often eradicate the negative message(s).

Here is one more witch message, which I received when I was in eighth grade music class in P.S. 6 in the Bronx. We were all to sing along with the teacher. As I recall, after class the teacher came up to me and told me that in the future I was to sit in the back of the room as I had no ear for music, and I was to be a "listener." When I was growing up in the Bronx there was no one in my immediate family, nor any relative or friend, who was musical or even taking music lessons. It was not until my forties that I got involved with music and took piano lessons. My teacher should have started with having me learn scales and distinguishing notes, but she did not. As a result, even at the end of five years of lessons, I could not tell her which of three notes she played on the piano was the highest! To continue, I do have a "big" voice and during the piano lesson time I actually took voice lessons for three years with an extraordinarily patient teacher. At the end of that time I could sing a Mozart aria, but only if I was listening to a recording! I stopped lessons when she was playing scales for me to sing, and she told me that I was singing the scales appropriately, but not in the correct octave! However, I did achieve that high for me of singing a Mozart aria.

Here are a few examples of witch messages:

- You'll never succeed.
- I despair that you will even find someone to marry you.
- How can you be so unfeeling and selfish?
- You never get anything right, do you?
- Why are you such a negative/mean/unloving/inconsiderate/sad/miserable/helpless/stupid/rebellious/ugly/disobedient/ignorant/impossible/selfish and uncaring/self-centered/ornery child? (Wow!)
- And, God will punish you for this, you'll see.

These are just a few examples, and the sad thing is that the speaker often feels that they are being helpful when they tell you this. My guess is that my eighth grade teacher felt that she was helping me by being realistic. (One remarkable (and reverse) aspect of this is telling a teacher that Johnny or Mary is much smarter than he/she appears to be. A teacher's response to that information is to *expect* higher and better performance from that student, which then becomes a reality. This has been tested.)

12.5 Andrea's Exercises and Change Processes

To give some idea of Andreas's work I cite the chapter headings of his two books: Book One—*Transforming Negative Self-talk* (2012): 1. Changing Location; 2. Changing Tempo and Locality; 3. Adding Music or a Song; 4. Talking to Yourself Positively; 5. Adding a Voice; 6. Auditory Perspective; 7. Starting Your Day; 8. Generalizations, Evaluations, Presuppositions, and Deletions; 9. Negative Messages and Positive Outcomes; 10. Asking Questions; 11. Transforming a Message. Book Two—*More Transforming Negative Self-talk* (2014a): 1. Joining With a Voice; 2. Retrieving and Clarifying Information; 3. Asking for the Positive Intent; 4. Putting it Together; 5. Listening for an Underlying Problem; 6. Making Use of a Voice's Special Abilities; 7. Using the Voice of a Trusted Friend; 8. Putting it Together—Again; 9. Putting it Together—in a Different Way; 10. Protecting Yourself From External Voices; 11. Not Talking Back; and 12. Not Silencing Your Inner Voice. In this section

I will briefly describe three interventions from each book. [Note: That three from Book One were also cited in Battino (2015).]

A. Changing Location of the Voice (Book One)

The negative voice that talks to us speaks to us from somewhere: inside our heads or bodies, or from outside somewhere. The basic idea in these interventions is to change the impact of the negative voice and its message(s) by making them disappear, minimizing their controlling characteristics, or even change the message(s) towards positive talk. In the last sense, it is even possible to *reframe* the messages.

In terms of location, is the voice coming from somewhere inside your body, or somewhere outside and from what location? If the voice is from outside, is it pointed towards or away from you or from some in between place? Now, notice what happens when you listen to that voice coming from a *different* location (inside or outside). Then, listen to that voice when it comes from a location that is *least disturbing* to you. When listening to the voice coming from inside your body, notice the location or site from which it is most disturbing, *and* least disturbing or troubling. You can also change the distance that the outside voice is coming from along with its location—notice what changes when you do this. When you have carried out these experiments you will realize that you actually have changed the location of the voice and its impact. With practice the ability to do this becomes easier.

The self-critical voice generally starts its statement with "I am ..." or "You are ..." This is an important distinction to consider. What happens when you change "I am ..." to "You are ..." or vice versa? That is, who is making the statement (is it you or someone else)? Have you incorporated the statement into your own self-image, or are you allowing someone else's ideas and opinions control you? Does the statement come with an image? Is the image of someone else or of something within you? You can change the location of the image and the image itself.

The volume of the speaking voice also has an effect. You can decrease the volume by moving the voice farther away, or using a "volume control" and just turning down the volume. What happens when you do this? As you rehearse all of these changes they will become more of your automatic thinking.

Andreas gives two cautions. The first has to do with the possibility that a change may make you feel worse. If this happens, respect this and change the voice back to the more comfortable level that existed before you made this change. The second is that the purpose of transforming negative self-talk is to convert the voice and its message to something that is more useful and supportive. It is not to eliminate it. This means that you can "talk" with the voice to find out its intent, and then decide as to whether you want to exist with it or eliminate it.

B. Adding Music or a Song (Book One)

It is well known that music can have profound effects on mood and emotions. People who have Alzheimer's disease or severe dementia have significantly impaired memories, yet they respond to music from their past, and can sing along and even dance to that music. Note that music is primarily processed in the right hemisphere of the brain for a right-handed person, and that this hemisphere does not process language. So, for a person without dementia but with a mood or emotional concern adding music or a song when they wish to bring about a change can be quite effective. They can ask themselves, "What kind of music would change my emotional state in an useful way?"

When you are in that disturbing mood, think of the meliorating music or song that will change that mood, hear that music or song, and *pair* it with the mood. Continue to hear the music and then think of a time when the mood was particularly disturbing. Notice what happens. Then do the same thing with other pieces of music until you find one (or more pieces) that shift your response in an useful manner. To condition yourself to respond to the troubling mood, think of a situation where this music would be helpful, enter that situation in your mind, and then recall the helping/healing music and listen to it. Adjust the volume and location of the music so that it is most helpful. Practicing this will make your musical response automatic.

Another way that can sometimes help when you are hearing troublesome messages in your mind is to "drown out" the voice with circus music or band music or other music that completely occupies your attention. Again, practicing this will make this kind of response automatic. Although I am not particularly fond of marching band music I have a friend for whom listening to this kind of music was his way of relaxing.

(While I think of it, I will mention that the sense of smell is our most primitive sense, that is, it is located in the primitive part of the brain. For this to help in troublesome situations you can think of the odors of a time in your life when you felt particularly loved and protected and safe and inhale deeply through your nose and let that remembered odor(s) carry you back to that time and place. If you can purchase that odor in some way (a sachet or perfume spray, for example), then use it during a stressful time.)

C. Talking Positively to Yourself (Book One)

This approach is an example of As-If behavior. Andreas poses this as, "For example, try saying the sentence, 'What else can I enjoy right now?' to yourself, and notice how it changes what you attend to, and how you feel in response …" He continues, "That sentence directs your attention toward what you can enjoy in the present moment, rather than the complaints and problems that so often occupy our attention and make us feel bad." Also, the word "else" in that sentence presupposes that you are already enjoying something. In terms of As-If this sentence gets you to consider acting (As-If!) in a different way. And, the word "enjoy" can be replaced by any other verb like: learn, see more clearly, understand, appreciate, do, create, etc.

Saying *affirmations* to yourself are a way of reframing how you perceive and feel about yourself. Here are some (the first four from Andreas):

- "I am healthy, happy, wise, and free."
- "I am surrounded by people who love me."
- "What else pleases me right now?"
- "What else is beautiful to me right now?"
- "I am feeling more relaxed/comfortable/capable/active."
- "I am ready to change something today."

The "Appreciate and Smile Exercise" has the person start with their eyes closed and imagining that they are in front of the door to their house, feeling the key in their hand, opening the door, and then asking them to "appreciate the door and smile." Then, continuing, they are asked to go around their home and appreciate and smile at everything they see and hear. This process can be repeated with appreciating and smiling with: family members, neighbors, acquaintances, strangers, and places they visit like office and school and shops. A wonderful healing and healthy suggestion is that they go inside their own bodies and appreciate and smile at all of their body parts!

Since noticing happy things *implies* feeling happy, another suggestion is for a person to look around their home (for example) and mentally say to themselves things like, "I am sitting on this happy chair. Over there is this happy table. And, here are the happy windows with their happy curtains." They can add to this whatever they wish, and also do this whenever they enter their real home. The mental exercise (and real experience) can be done for 5–10 minutes every day for a while. (It might even become a habit!)

Another As-If way of changing behavior was developed by Nardone and Portelli (2005, p. 73). It is similar to the Miracle Question. Their directions are:

> During the following weeks, I'd like you to ask yourself this question. Every day, in the morning, question yourself: "What would I do differently today if I no longer had this problem, or if I had recovered from my problem? Among all the things that come to your mind, choose the smallest, most minimal but concrete thing, and put it into practice. Every day, choose a small but concrete thing as if you had already overcome your problem, and voluntarily put it into practice. Every day choose something different.

There are a number of significant words in this set of instructions: "smallest," "concrete," "voluntarily," "choose something different," and the action phrase of "put it into practice." (Recall that in guiding changes in your client's behavior you are endeavoring to convert their "I can't" to "I won't," which is the conversion of involuntary to voluntary behavior.)

The "Three Gifts" exercise[1] was developed by Silvester (2010, pp. 229–231) and he comments that positive psychologists have found that over a seven-day period their approach was more effective in raising the mood of people with depression than Prozac (Seligman, 2003). The directions for this exercise are:

Each evening for one week look back over your day and select three positive things that have happened and write them down. Also, please write down how you were responsible for those "gifts" occurring.

This is another variant of As-If procedures. It is also a solution-focused exercise. People will find that their ability to find three "gifts" each day grows as they actively look for them daily. In a sense, the magic of Silvester's exercise is in the developing *expectation* of the person finding gifts in their daily lives. The Three Gifts idea can be easily expanded to: (1) Gratitude: find three opportunities on any given day to thank somebody for something beyond everyday pleasantries; (2) Savoring: choose two or three things each day to savor—these can be food, Nature, family or friends, and anything you interact with; (3) Kindness: find a way to do an act of kindness every day with no thought of personal gain, and also with some inconvenience or cost to you. These are easy activities, and yet they can have a profound effect on how you feel about yourself.

D. Transforming a Message (Book One)

This brilliant way of transforming a message was developed by Melanie Davis (a therapist in the UK) and has been further developed by Andreas (2012, pp. 107–116). Here are the elements of the approach (pp. 109–110):

1 Presuppose that what your client has been saying to himself is positive and useful, but has been badly misunderstood.
2 Divide the sentence into two or more parts.
3 Use *auditory ambiguity* to find a different meaning in the same sounds (or similar sounds) that is more positive, enjoyable, humorous, or even nonsensical.
4 Use a different intonation and inflection that is cheerful, playful, and humorous, instead of the serious or unpleasant one in the original statement.
5 The meaning of the message is changed, but no attempt is made to change the intensity of the client's feeling response.

This is illustrated in what follows.

Let's begin with the message, "I'm no good." This transforms to the two sentences that you ask the client to say. They are, "I am" and "I *know* good." Ask the client to say these two sentences aloud and with conviction, and several times. They can be written large and with a heavy black permanent marker on a blank piece of paper with the second sentence below the first. The client keeps this as an "anchor" for the transformation.

Here is another one, "Don't think I will sleep tonight." This becomes, "Don't think" and I *will* sleep tonight." A variant of "I'll never be able to sleep" becomes: "I'll never!" and "Be able to sleep." Or to: "I will? Never!" and "Be able to sleep." Some additional pairings follow:

- No one likes me. "No! one likes me." or "*Know*—one likes me!"
- Something is wrong with me. "Something is ... row with me" or "Some think strong with me."
- I'm so inadequate. "I'm so IN! Adequate!"
- It's not fair. "It is! Not fair?" or "It's not fare!" (food) or "It's a nutta fair." (With an Italian accent.)
- I'm not worthy. "I'm noteworthy" or "I am noteworthy." Or "I am!—Not worthy?"
- No one will marry me. "NO! One **will** marry me" or "Know! ONE will marry me."

This kind of verbal transformation is also a reframing in the sense that the client is getting a different perspective on the message that has been troubling him/her. The affirmations anchor the change in what they had believed about themselves. Repetition in various voices and ways reinforces the message. Also, writing the new message boldly on a white board or newsprint or project paper provides a permanent visual and solid reminder for the change.

Transforming the troubling message is a confusion technique, almost along the lines of the *inclusivity* method. You accept the message and then in an oxymoronic manner convert it to its opposite.

E. Joining with a Voice (Book Two)

An internal voice that troubles you is a recorded voice of difficult times in relationships with others in your personal history. It is important to know that if you fight or argue with or attempt to eliminate that voice, that it will usually fight back (just as it would have done in the real world). Andreas comments (p. 12), "But if you take steps to befriend a troublesome internal voice and ally yourself with it, you can develop a positive relationship with it, and begin to move toward resolution of your differences." That is, this would be an useful first step in terms of really listening to it and understanding how it functions. (This approach is in line with Stephen Levine's recommendation of *not fighting* the cancer that is part of you, but working with all of your body's resources in minimizing the effects of the cancer as you strengthen and enhance your own immune system. That is, "wars" on various diseases appear to invite resistance.)

One interesting approach discussed by Andreas is to *exaggerate* what the voice says as this paradoxical method often results in diminishing your own feeling response to it. (Note that exaggeration of a symptom is a common Gestalt Therapy technique. You keep exaggerating the symptom until it vanishes under its own weight.)

Andreas also writes (p. 16),

> Another way to deepen your understanding of what a voice is communicating is to discover the underlying assumption or attitude in what it is saying, and exaggerate that instead of the voice itself. ... If you exaggerate this underlying assumption, you can often elicit a useful change in your response.

In a sense, exaggeration weakens the message and voice.

F. Asking for the Positive Intent (Book Two)

One of the questions that NLP practitioners frequently ask of a client is to *find the intent* (positive or negative) associated with a particular behavior that the client wishes to change. It is therefore helpful to ask any voice for its positive intent since the answer can be useful. You do not need to know much about the origins of the voice, just that it has been there for some time and has had an impact on how you feel and act. Andreas states that if you keep asking about a negative intent, you will always eventually find a positive one. Once you know the positive intent behind the voice, that is something you can obviously agree with. This changes your relationship with the voice. At this point you can work together with the voice to change what the voice says and how it says it so that its behavior becomes aligned with its positive intent. Then you can negotiate with the voice to change that positive intent to something that you would like to hear, and that continues its goal of helping you.

G. Using the Voice of a Trusted Friend (Book Two)

Once you know the positive intent of the voice, Andreas indicates that there are three different aspects of this: (1) the positive intent itself, that is, what the voice wants to accomplish; (2) the desire to communicate this positive intent to someone else; and (3) the voice's implicit desire to be acknowledged and appreciated for its positive intent (communicating this to the voice satisfies its need for appreciation). Now, having the voice use the voice of a trusted friend will make you happy to listen to it. The steps for doing this are (pp. 77–79):

1   *Select the Friend.* Think of a trusted friend of the same sex as the voice, and of someone you know who cares for you. (This person would listen to whatever you had to say.)
2   *Listen to the Friend's Voice.* You need to know his/her tonality, volume, tempo, etc.
3   *Ask the Troublesome Voice to Adopt this Tonality.* That is, would you be willing to use this tonality, and know that I am only asking you to try an alternative?
4   *Testing.* If the voice says no, back up and clear up any misunderstanding. If the voice says yes, have it try out that voice.
5   *Thank the Voice.* Sincerely thank the voice for doing this.
6   *Adjustments.* After listening to the voice (in 4) suggest changes to get it just right.
7   *Rehearsal and Testing.* The testing is done by imagining a future situation in which you might want this voice to speak to you, and then notice what happens spontaneously. If it is the trusted voice, then good. If it is not, you need to go back and check with the voice.
8   *Congruence Check.* This is done by asking if any part of you has any objections or concerns about these changes, and then working through them.
9   *Satisfy Objections.* This can be done by adjusting the changes, reframing them, or working with the contexts so that they do not interfere with important outcomes.

H. Comments on Andreas's "Transforming Negative Self-Talk"

The previous material is an introduction to Andreas's work, and contains enough information for you to use a number of these ways of transforming witch messages. I have already used a number of these methods with clients and they do seem to be a bit magical in how rapidly they can bring about changes. In this sense, let me quote Andreas (2014, p. 54), "Change does not have to take long. Change can be very quick. You may need a lot of little quick changes to get to an eventual outcome, but I believe that all change is almost instantaneous." Wow! Consider that reframing, the Miracle Question, As-If methods, inclusivity, and metaphoric work, et al., all appear to work as Eureka! discoveries, transcendental moments, and religious conversions. When you see the light …

12.6 Healing Language Scenarios

There are some 68 scenarios for using healing language in my book (Battino, 2010). Their format is: a title, patient says, closed response, open response, hostile response, and empathic response. (Scenarios may not contain all of these responses.) Appendix B in the 2010 book, pp. 207–209, contains brief versions of 13 scenarios that are the ones most likely to be used by health professionals. To give you some idea of the scope of these scenarios, here are the titles of these 13: Lung Cancer; Cancer in Remission; Palliative Care; Inoperable Tumor; Giving a Prognosis; Patient Died in the OR; Radical Prostatectomy; Bone Marrow Transplant; Pancreatic Cancer and End-of-Life; AIDS and End-of-Life; Brain Death; Pain—Discussion Pain Control; and Child With Cancer. In the following I will give the short scenarios for six circumstances from the previous list (with the long version of one of them), and the full scenarios for three scenarios for non-medical circumstances. (Scenario and page numbers are from Battino (2010).)

Scenario 1— Lung Cancer—A 40-year-old man who is a fitness fanatic, except for his smoking, develops lung cancer. *Response*: It must be very hard to accept a serious illness when you feel so fit (p. 207).

Scenario 2—Cancer in Remission—There is a significant chance it will recur in the next few years. *Response*: It must be awful for you to be continually worrying about a recurrence (p. 207).

Scenario 11—Giving a Prognosis—Test results have come in and the patient has asked for a prognosis. *Response*: I can tell you what the statistics say. Everyone is different. I know this is almost impossibly hard for you, but I will stick with you and help in any way I can. If you push me for a number now, I would give you a range of a few months to several years (p. 207).

Scenario 24—Pancreatic Cancer and End-of-Life—A 72-year-old patient is told that he has pancreatic cancer, which has metastasized. *Response*: This is serious since the cancer has metastasized and there are no treatments. You may wish to take advantage of the local hospice program—they are very good at keeping you comfortable and helping with family. You can call on me any time and I will be available (p. 208).

Scenario 33—Brain Death—A blood clot has broken through and the patient is brain dead. Telling the family. *Response*: I don't know how to tell you this. The surgery went well, but a clot somehow formed and broke loose and entered his/her brain. He/she is effectively brain dead. I'll stay with you. Let me take you to him/her. I know this impossibly hard (p. 208).

Scenario 53—Child With Cancer—A. Telling Parents Response: The tests are in and I am very sorry to tell you she/he has cancer. It is treatable with a good prognosis. The treatments will be hard on you and _____ (name child). We will give you all the support and help we can. *B. Telling Child*

Response: You have a very serious illness. We know how to treat it and we are sure you will come through this well. Some of the treatments may make you feel bad, but we have lots of good medicines to help, and your parents can stay with you.

Scenario 54—Child, Carcinoma of the Leg, Amputation—A formerly very active 12-year-old boy has been diagnosed with a carcinoma in his leg. This has progressed to the point where the only option to save his life appears to be to amputate the leg above the knee. After that operation, chemotherapy is an option.

1   *Empathy*—This can be hard on anyone, and you've already been through so much. We have three doctors who agree that this is the best thing to do for you. Fortunately, you're a very strong boy—you'll do well with the surgery. This will really fix it. There'll be some hard work getting used to an artificial leg. I'm sure you're going to be surprised at how much you'll be able to do afterwards. How are you feeling now? Any questions?

2   *Healing*—I can tell you're thinking I won't be able to do this and that, and it'll hurt. We can control any pain or discomfort—you've been through a lot already and you know that. I can show you pictures and introduce you to boys who have been through this. You'll be surprised at how much you'll be able to do. But, right now, what's going on inside of you? (p. 166).

Scenario 60—Losing a Game—16-year-old Ellen is on the girls' school soccer team—they've just lost an important game.

1   *Empathy*—You look so sad. Do you want to talk about it now? That was a tough one to lose. I could tell how hard you were all playing. Can I have a hug?

2   *Healing*—You were really doing well. It's hard to lose by one goal, especially an important game like this one. I could tell you were playing your best—I enjoyed watching you out there. You seemed to be enjoying just playing, too. I liked the way you played as a team—you work well together. Still, it's hard to lose sometimes. How are you feeling? But, right now I'd like to give you a great big hug. Okay? (p. 170).

Scenario 62—Spilling a Glass of Milk—Little Ellen has spilled a glass of milk all over the table.

1   *Empathy*—Well, you're improving. That was just a little spill and you got your napkin there right away.

2   *Healing*—Don't worry, honey, it's just a little milk. I'm glad nothing broke. You are getting better and better and bigger and bigger. It's hard

using a real glass. I'm so proud of you. Here, let's clean it up together (p. 170).

Scenario 67—Supervisor/Employee—An employee has messed up an important assignment. The supervisor/boss is angry about this.

1 *Empathy 1*—You must feel awful about this. You knew how important it was. I don't know what went wrong, and I want no excuses. Fix it up. You can have some help if you need it.
2 *Empathy 2*—You must know that this isn't acceptable. You're generally a very good worker. What went wrong with this assignment? We can fix it up, but I need to know what happened so this doesn't happen again. Okay?
3 *Healing*—You must know this is unacceptable. You are usually so reliable. What's been going on? Do you need more help? You know we need to meet deadlines. This can probably be fixed. You look awful. You know, there are a lot of ways to learn—messing up is one of them. I expect you to learn from this and do better. You have a good head—use it, please (p. 170).

If you are interested in learning more about the use of scenarios, language for healing, and related matters, please see my book on this subject. The footnote[2] on this page contains the chapter headings in that book.

12.7 Reframing and Healing Language

A long time ago I did a workshop on reframing and there are some things I did then that I will describe here since they may be useful today. In that era (before PowerPoint and projection systems for lectures) overhead projectors and slides were the devices of choice. I had the university artist draw colorful frames of various kinds on the cardboard frames for these slides. In addition to patterns there were faces and animals on the frames. I had the participants in the workshop pick up a frame and walk around looking through it at the other people similarly walking around. Then, they traded these frames and continued their wandering. This was done for six or so changes. At that time I did not have a large mirror available or I would have had each person also look at themselves in a mirror. The participants quickly got the message of how a frame can change their perception of each other. If I did this again in a group setting or with an individual client, I would have one or more mirrors of different sizes available. Not only can a picture framer change the impact of a painting or photo or other art work, but we also can change our perception of how we view others and ourselves in this active physical (kinesthetic) manner.

In f2f therapy we use words and verbal images and suggestions to reframe. NLP introduced a linguistic structure that is relevant to negative self-talk and reframing. It is called *complex equivalence*, which is two statements that are equivalent in a person's model or perception of the world. There is an implied causal connection between the two statements. In the following examples note the negative self-talk.

- I've developed this cancer ... I must have done something wrong some time.
- I got AIDS and I don't know why ... God has given up on me—He doesn't love me.
- I am having so much pain now ... Am I being punished for something?
- When my husband looks at me that way ... I just know that he has just given up hope *or* that he doesn't love me any more.
- He acts in such different ways now ... he must really be crazy.

When you examine these paired statements they appear to be foolish and even nonsensical. Why would anyone believe them and draw these conclusions? Yet, I think you would all recognize that not only do people you know make such irrational connections, but you have likely done so in the past.

A *content or meaning reframe* can be done with a complex equivalence to "challenge" the connected assertion. That is, this effectively changes certainty to choice. Here are some possible reframes to the above statements:

- There are known substances that are carcinogens, but your type of cancer is not related to one of them. The fact is that we do not know how a cancer like that starts. And, it was certainly nothing that you did.
- You know that a loving God loves all of His children, and that He would certainly not give AIDS to anyone. Listen, no matter what some unthinking religious people out there say, God loves you and I love you.
- The pain you are feeling occurs in many of my patients who have this kind of cancer. It is the cancer that is causing the pain—no one is punishing you. There are many things we can do working together to make you more comfortable.
- You can't read people's minds from the way that they are looking at you. The best way to know what he is thinking is just to ask him directly, "When you look at me, as you are doing now, I just do not know what you are thinking. Please tell me."
- I have observed many people and have been amazed at all of the different ways they behave that make no sense to me. I find them endlessly interesting, and I appreciate and am curious about them.

Simple verbal reframing changes the "frame" or way or perceiving whatever it is that is reframed as in:

- It must have taken a lot of courage to talk today to me so openly about what has been bothering you.
- Clients like you have taught me a great deal.
- Cancer is not a sentence, it is a word.
- You know that it is okay to withhold anything you don't want to tell me.
- Pain is only a signal. Please let me know about any changes. Okay?
- You're right in saying that a prognosis is just an educated guess. So, here is my best guess. You're the kind of person to prove me wrong.
- You may not believe this, but to have gone through what you have been telling me about and still keep going is remarkable. Thank you for sharing.

There is another kind of reframing that is called *context reframing*, and this is based on the idea that every behavior is useful somewhere and in some circumstance. The question then to consider it, "In what context or circumstance would this particular behavior be of value to you?" Several examples follow:

- Family and relationships are what it is all about, aren't they?
- If you can't cry/joke/laugh/yell/get angry/tell the truth/fall apart/be yourself or come together here, where else can you do it? Think now about some other places.
- Sometimes a good place to feel lost is in a crowd; and a good place to find yourself is with other people.
- Where would you be the most comfortable in sharing what you told me? Would it be with your wife/husband/children/friend/boss?
- You know that you don't have to be sick or miserable or depressed to: ask for what you need/be hugged/pray/review your life/smell the roses/enjoy a sunset or sunrise/have some quiet time/eat a reasonable amount of something special.

I heard about a man who turned around the ambiance of the nursing home he became in charge of by stating loudly in the day room where the residents gathered to seemingly vegetate by saying, "It this a *waiting* room or a *living* room?" This was followed by many ways of involving the residents in the daily activities of the place and giving them responsibilities like caring for plants in their rooms, and leading some of the communal activities. I may be repetitious here in stating that I have found that almost all of the clinical demonstrations I have witnessed at meetings could be characterized as reframing (no matter the orientation of the presenter).

12.8 Two Concluding Sets of Healing Activities

A. Bernie Siegel's Questions for People with Life-Challenging Diseases

1 Why me?
2 Why now?
3 Why this particular disease?
4 Why am I getting better or worse at this time?
5 At this time, what do I sense will help me?

When you are working with someone who has a life-challenging disease, the answers they give to these questions guide you (and them) in what to do next. Many people feel that it is something they have done that resulted in this disease—once openly verbalized then this belief can be discussed and even challenged. It does need to be openly conscious for any action to be taken. Question 4 lets you and them know their current status. Also, 1 and 4 are related to either a person's belief system or to the treatments they are having or have had. And, 5 provides an opening for a guided imagery session and/or further explorations.

B. Bernie Siegel's Four Drawings

Bernie has done a lot of work with art therapy in terms of having his patients make drawings. If *you* interpret what you see someone draw, then you are imposing *your* beliefs about symbolism and content. It is important for the artist to give meanings and interpretations to the drawings or parts of them. Elicit *their* meanings. Here are the four types of drawings:

1 Make a drawing of you in your current state, that is how you feel and look now.
2 Make a drawing about any treatments you are having and/or have received.
3 Make a drawing of how you would look after you are well and all of this is behind you.
4 Finally, make a drawing of how you got from (1) to (3).

Although this set of four drawings was originally designed for people who have life-challenging diseases, the same set of four can be used for people who have psychological difficulties. (Please note that these steps parallel Rossi's moving/mirroring hands four-step approach to doing psychotherapy.)

Notes

1 This exercise is strongly connected to Pennebaker's exercise for students (Pennebaker, 1997; Pennebaker and Chung, 2007)). It simply involves having students (generally freshmen) write for 20 minutes daily for two weeks about their emotions. They found that this exercise significantly helped the students adjust to college life.

2 Chapter titles in *Healing Language* follow: 1. Introduction to Healing and Hope-filled Communication; 2. Rapport—Connecting with People; 3. Healing Language Forms; 4. Witch Messages; 5. Reframing and Healing; 6. Healing Contact; 7. Robert Buckman, M.D.'s Work; 8. Healing Language for Medical Doctors; 9. Responses from Patients, Caregivers, Nurses, and Physicians; 10. Healing Communication for Nurses; 11. Healing Language With Friends and Relatives; 12. Children; 13. Healing Words for Institutions; 14. Healing Words—Rituals and Ceremonies; 15. Iserson's Grave Words; 16. Some Final Healing Words.

13 Case Study 7

Jennifer, Anxiety, Manzanita Beach, and Jesus[1]

a single leaf moves
trembled by a passing breeze
then slowly settles

R (RUBIN):   Is there anything you would like to work on this afternoon, something in your life you would like to change?

J (JENNIFER):   My stress. My anxiety.

R: And, I will protect your privacy. This is your time. Erickson liked to start
with something like, "Please don't tell me anything you don't want to tell
me." Perhaps I can get a little background. How long has this stress been
going on?

J: The really bad stress in … the last four or five months.

R: Four or five months. Perhaps there is something in your mind that would
let me know how it started back then? You don't have to tell me about it.
This is more like secret therapy. I really see myself more as a guide than
someone who does things to people. … More about that time, perhaps
later. So, we can now find some way so you will be more relaxed and calm
about your life. Okay? And, maybe at some time I may want to make
some comments to the audience. Would that be okay?

J: Yes. (She reached forward and touched my hands.)

R: In a strange way my hands are a bit colder than yours. I may be more
stressed than you are. (She laughed.) I notice your name is Jennifer. May
I call you that?

J: Yes.

R: One of the things I do with a client when I feel stuck is to literally switch
seats with them. Then I play you and you play me. When that happens
I sometimes play you tougher than you would play me. And you have to
help me! That's one way of going about this that might work.

J: Huh.

R: One of the things I do a great deal with people is guided imagery. Do you
know what that process is?

J: Yes.

R: I am thinking more of using that at this time for it is a way of protecting you more, if you will.

J: Yes.

R: In my experience everyone who goes inside themselves goes into some level of trance. I never worry about how deep that might be. If I were a surgeon, I would worry more about that. But just enough, okay?

J: Okay.

R: When I do guided imagery work there are three things I always ask about that would be helpful. The first thing I ask about is, "Have you had any experience in doing relaxation or meditation or self-hypnosis or something like that, Jennifer?"

J: Yes. I have done a little bit of that.

R: What about meditation?

J: Yes. I have done a little bit of that.

R: And, how do you get into a meditative state?

J: Sometimes I close my eyes, lay down on a mat and relax.

R: Do you sometimes do things like count numbers? I find that a lot of my clients do that.

J: Yes. I do a little bit of that.

R: So, would just paying attention to your breathing work? That works with most people.

J: Yes, I can do that.

R: Now, just getting back to the idea of hypnosis. I have a simplified definition about what hypnosis is. Any time your attention is so focused on something that the world around you disappears, then you are in some trance state. So, any time you are so focused on something like reading or music, then you are in a kind of trance. It is nothing mysterious, we do this all of the time. It is not a kind of Svengali kind of thing.

J: (Laughs)

R: The second thing that is going to be useful is something I call a Safe Haven. Do you have a place you would go to within your mind, that is real or imaginary, that is safe and secure, where you would be comfortable, and maybe even a learning place?

J: Hm.

R: It could be a wilderness or a lake or a beach or …

J: Yes, a beach. Manzanita Beach on the Oregon coast. It is near my office.

R: Wonderful, since a few years ago my wife and I drove all of the way down the Oregon coast and stopped there. That was a great experience.

J: Yes.

R: The third thing that is going to be helpful and useful is: do you have an internal feeling or sense that there is something or someone who can help you with this stuff that has been troubling you, and would make them all go away?

J: Hm.

R: In my experience, people choose things like healing hands or healing light, or religious people use someone like Jesus or the Holy Spirit or God.

J: Well, I'm religious and Catholic.

R: Would the Holy Spirit work for you?

J: Yes.

R: Good. One other thing. You were so nice at the beginning to reach out and hold my hand. I wonder if some time during the session it would be okay to reach out and hold your hand?

J: Sure. (She reaches out and touches my hand.)

R: That's part of the process. So, let me say something about my volunteer work. For about 25 years I have worked with a group of people who have serious ailments, and guided imagery has proven to be quite helpful for that. It was started by the Simontons many years ago. It's become the standard way of doing those things. I've had a lot of experience doing this kind of thing.

J: Sure.

R: I'm really glad that it is not something else. ... So, it is probably quite manageable.

J: (Nods.)

R: And I may even ask you now, how surprised you would be if this all disappeared in one little session this afternoon?

J: Hm. Okay. I'll try.

R: Let me share my philosophy with you. I always have hope and I believe in miracles. My work has been with people who have real serious diseases.

J: Hm.

R: I've seen people walk out of hospice. That is, they have "graduated" from hospice.

J: Hm.

R: So, things like that happen. [Seeding a "miraculous" change.] Now, let's see if you can find a way to be a bit more comfortable. Okay?

J: Hm.

R: And, being comfortable, closing your eyes, if that is okay, or just looking off into the distance. As I said earlier, you can now just pay attention to your breathing. Just noticing each breath as it goes in and comes out. With each inhale chest and belly softly rising, and then with each exhale all of those muscles just relaxing. Just one breath at a time. One heart-beat at a time. Softly, easily, simply. And, occasionally Jennifer, a stray thought may wander through. Notice it, thank it for being there, and go back to ... And, if I don't use just the right words or images this after-noon, please feel free to change them so that they are just the right words and images you need to help you today. You can notice the way that your hands are on your thighs, the way that your feet make contact with the floor. This breath and the next one. And, within your mind now you can just drift off to Manzanita Beach. And, you know that place very well, do you not? A wonderful place, yes, a wonderful place. The sounds of the ocean … sand. I don't know the particular place where you are. Yet, you know. There are some of those outcrops of rocks there, are there not? And, then those big white fluffy clouds floating around. And, then there are the waves coming in, sliding up the sand. And then just sinking into the sand and going back out into the water, the surf. And the wind. Just warm enough. Maybe. And just the breeze.

And, now something interesting is going to happen. Continuing to breathe calmly, easily, naturally. And somewhere near you is the Holy Spirit. And, the Holy Spirit is knowledgeable, powerful, a healer. A great sense of love, compassion, and sensitivity. And the Holy Spirit is coming a bit closer. You can sense His presence, can you not? And, in some way, the Holy Spirit is able to reach out and touch you. You can feel that contact, that sense of connection with the Holy Spirit. To the Holy Spirit. The sounds, the sky, the surroundings. Almost the whole way out to the universe. And, the Holy Spirit knows just where within you to send His loving compassionate knowledge. Just those places within your body to send, what?, a calming, a sense of peace, a sense of self, of knowing deeply who you are. From your toes all the way to the hair on top of your head. An inner sense of yes, it's okay, I'm okay. Yes. That, somehow, with this contact with the Holy Spirit that whatever it is that had been troubling you has just somehow been cleansed and washed away.

Just like the way the waves roll up the beach, footsteps, birds, markings on the sands, and the sand becomes just sand again, clean, calm, ready for … maybe somebody walking on the beach. Maybe for whatever is coming next. Maybe someone with a dog walking, perhaps, the dog running into the water and running along the beach. Leaving little footprints, just as you have in your life. Many footprints, and it's good to know that … what? Sort of like leaving your mark on the world, leaving your impressions. And it's good to know your footprints are there … Calmly, easily, naturally. One breath at a time, one heartbeat.

And, I am going to ask you at this time if it is okay to hold your hand. I'll put out my hand, Jennifer, and you put out your hand and we make contact. [At this point I have extended my hand towards her, but she does not respond. Her hand is tilted forward and she appears to be in a deep trance.] If it is okay. And if it is not okay, now, then at this time just stay in the presence of the Holy Spirit. [I withdraw my hand.] And, in some interesting way, somehow, I do not know how, the Holy Spirit is able to reach into your essence, your soul, your mind, your very life, and it may be that there is some wiring that needs to be rearranged, or arranged with different connections. It may be that some memories may be useful to modify, or changed, or to forget. And the Holy Spirit knows in its infinite wisdom and compassion with love, just exactly what to do and how to do that, how to rearrange. And also how to send that into your body, every atom, every molecule, every cell, every tissue, every bone, every organ, so that they can sense changes, re-energizing, reorganizing, renovating, reconnecting, in a way that would be most helpful and most effective for you at this time.

This breath, and the next one. And the Holy Spirit having helped you at this time, and done His work, in this time of your need, to bring about those changes that would be and are most helpful and realistic to you at this time, slowly withdraws. For, as you know, He has much more work to do.

And, there is that cloud floating up there. Wonderful. Waves rolling up the beach. Perhaps some gulls making their cries in the background. A soft breeze blowing through the bushes and grass at the end of the beach. And as you walk along the beach now, calmly, easily, naturally, you are probably aware that your memory is somewhat like a recording machine. So that whatever ideas, images, thoughts, words, that you have heard today, your experiences, and having been in the presence of and made contact with the Holy Spirit, He will be with you whenever you need Him and as you need Him. Perhaps, finding a quiet place where you can pay attention to your breathing, and thinking back, you will be able to relive and re-experience again this time, your time, with the Holy Spirit. A smile, a touch, joy, the moon in the morning, and the sun at sunset, peace and quiet.

And, I want to thank you Jennifer for your attention, your trust, your confidence, and whenever you are ready, perhaps, take a deep breath or two, blink your eyes, stretch a bit, just come back to this room here and now. Thank You. Wow! [Long pause. She returns, and we both smile at each other.] One of my experiences that goes with something like this is that you will generally remember [She reaches down for a tissue at this time.] some of the things that I said, some of the things that had transpired. So, what typically happens when people get into these really relaxed states is that sometime later you will remember parts of what happened, and forget others. [Pauses—many of them throughout—are not indicated above.]

J: This is, yes. Thank you.

R: Yes. Thank you. When you get into this again there are some things you can just reach out and grab. And sometime later my voice comes back with you again. Okay?

J: [Nods yes.]

R: Yes. So this is your time now. Anything more you want to do or ask about?

J: There are tears coming to my eyes. [Has issue in hand.] Thank you. [Reaches out with both hands to hold my hands.] My hands are so cold. Thank you.

R: Thank you.

J: I have a slight cold. [Smiles happily.]

R: One of the things I've become aware of that is important is something I learned from the NLP people, and that is about anchoring. That is, providing some way of providing a physical reminder of what's happened. And, perhaps with some sense of forethought, I have a little gift for you. Which, surprisingly, may be very appropriate. I'm going to reach into my pocket here and bring out the kind of stone that you might have found on Manzanita Beach. I'd like you to have that. [I give it to her. This is a small smooth black stone.]

J: Thank you.

R: So, that whenever you feel that you need another little bit of taking care of yourself, that will be with you. [She takes stone, and holds it in both hands.]

J: Thank you. Thank you very much.

R: Would it be okay now to find out if anyone in the audience has some comments or questions? Is that okay with you?

J: Yes.

R: And, if they ask something that you don't want to answer, that's what I am here for. Okay? [Always protect the volunteer.]

J: Yes. [We turn towards the audience.]

R: So, we're turning our chairs a bit towards the audience. I do not use diagnoses, but if I am forced to use one it is that you are "temporarily troubled." So, I might say to Jennifer—"You are temporarily troubled, and let's go on from there." [Jennifer laughs.]

J: I like that.

R: Let's listen to the words. "Temporarily" sets the stage and "troubled" is important. If your clients have "problems," those are big things, and they might spend three weeks telling you their sad stories and all about them! My clients have "troubles" or "concerns" or things that "bother" them. And they are amenable to being helped in that way. [Jennifer is nodding yes all through this.]

R: [Question about the healing helper.] I always ask the client what it is that they feel or sense inside them that is going to help them. That is *their* choice, and I am going to use *their* imagery. If my client wants something spiritual, then I work with them. A number of my clients have wanted Jesus to help them. I recall a client who was very religious who had cancer. Jesus helped her in these sessions. But, one day she said to me that Jesus was not enough. I asked what else she needed. She told me that it would help to have Native Americans, Indians, track down the cancer cells and ride round and round them, and just kill them and get rid of them with their arrows and tomahawks! So, that's what we did: at the beginning of each session I would ask her who she wanted to help her today. Sometimes it was Jesus, sometimes the Native Americans, and sometimes both. This was her choice. It is essential to work within the belief system of your client.

R: Any other comments?

QUESTION FROM AUDIENCE: [About making contact holding hands.]

R: Thank you. Yes. You have to follow the lead of your client. I put my hand out and your hands did not move at all. I followed along with that and withdrew my hand.

J: Yes.

R: One important thing about holding hands is that when do that my hand is passive. [Holding hands with Jennifer now.]

J: Like this.

R: Yes. I'm not going to grab your hand and caress it! Passive. [Jennifer laughs.]

J: Like this.

R: I do this within a guided imagery session along with using the word "somehow," which is a magic word, and say that you would get whatever you need now from me and *through* [another magic word] me. As an example, working with someone who had cancer, I indicate that my body does not have cancer, and that my immune system is working. So, my immune system is teaching and training theirs via the contact so that all of the information they need to make their immune system more effective and more efficient and more powerful in eliminating all of these crazy cells can be transferred. That is, *somehow* from me and *through me*. [Still holding hands.]

J: I didn't want to hold your hand. When I was on the beach I was holding Jesus's hand. I was just in that moment on the beach. It wasn't that I didn't want to hold your hand …

R: That's fine. I am not going to compete with Jesus! [Audience laughs. Coming to the end of the session.] Jennifer, may I ask one question? [OK] Are you feeling okay now?

J: Yes.

R: Great. Thank you. [End of session.]

[After the session was over and I was in the lobby getting ready to go to another session, Jennifer came up to me with the smooth stone in her hand that I had given her. She had a permanent marker and asked me to sign the stone! Although I had given her one of my business cards with my contact information on it, and told her that I would be delighted to hear from her, she never did make contact. She left smiling ...]

Commentary on Session

Guided imagery for psychotherapy embodies Erickson's *utilization principle* of using the client's own experiences and life. In effect, they are telling you what will work as a change agent for them! It also incorporates the concept of As-If behavior in the sense that the client is immersed in (and living through) their own imagery about what it is that has brought them to therapy. And, using carefully chosen vague language throughout, you are giving the client permission to fill in details reflecting their own lives and reality. This last idea is the essence of the power of hypnosis to change clients' behaviors and thoughts about themselves by incorporating and inserting open-ended suggestions. Clients always know (better than us) the realistic constraints on their lives, and hypnosis allows them to access and utilize these realities.

This clinical demonstration also illustrates the use of " secret therapy." That is, working with a client when you only have minimal information about what it is that troubles them. Please note that the only information I had about Jennifer at the beginning of the session was that she had been experiencing anxiety and stress for several months, and wanted to get over that. I did not have a long or detailed history about what help she wanted. At one time it was thought that a detailed history was needed before doing therapy, and before that time it also seemed that testing of various types was needed before starting therapeutic work. (There are, of course, circumstances when it might be useful to have a client take a "standard" test for depression.)

A few years ago I gave a presentation to a hypnosis group about what I called the "Yenta Syndrome." Wikipedia which gives two definitions for Yenta: (1) "Yenta or Yenta is a Yiddish designation for a woman who is a gentlewoman or noblewoman coming from the Yiddish translation of yenta to genteel/gentle." and (2) "The Yiddish name 'Yenta' derives from a word meaning 'gentle' or 'noble' but it has come to refer to a woman who is a gossip or a busybody ... In the age of Yiddish theater, it started referring to a *busybody or gossipmonger*." Currently, the italicized part of (2) is the common meaning of the word, and is the one that I am using here. I believe it would be safe to say that therapists are people who may be more curious about others than the normal population. Just what is going in their brain right now, why are they *really* here, and what kind of life have they led?

Psychoanalysis dominated most of the twentieth century, and how could the "analyst" analyze a client without extensive knowledge about their thinking and lives? So, they spent a great deal of time gathering information going back many years since they believed that the origins of current behavior was in early difficulties or traumas. A reasonable interpretation of their activities is that they were "Yentas" as described in the second definition above. This is relevant to the idea of doing "secret therapy." So, although it is useful to have information about the client and his/her history and the history of the presenting concerns, the questions are: (1) how much information do you really need to guide a client to the changes that are realistic and helpful and desirable to them; and (2) is it possible to provide such guidance with *only knowing* that they are currently troubled and hurting and seeking ways out of their stuckness? Many experienced therapists are good at eliciting minimal information. Others (like me) generally prefer to use a variety of what might be described as generic secret therapy approaches.

A brief list of them is: (1) guided imagery; (2) the Miracle Question; (3) Rossi's moving (or mirroring) hands approach; (4) acting As-If the change(s) had already occurred (as deciding to be happy); (5) the crystal ball approach where the client looks back from the future and tells you what they did to bring about their desired change(s); (6) Cheek's ideomotor finger signaling where the client goes back to the time their difficulty (or difficulties) started and are asked if it is okay now to *not respond* or react that way any more; (7) ambiguous function assignments where the client is persuaded to undertake some task or experience with the implication that by doing it they will discover needed understandings or changes; and (8) a variant of the Gestalt Therapy Two-Chair approach wherein the client carries out the two-person or two-part or two-reaction dialogue within themselves. One plus of doing secret therapy for therapists is that of not getting involved in and with the traumas and emotional states of their clients. That is, who needs to listen to all of that misery day in and day out? This does not mean that you cannot empathize with your clients and be there with them 100% in ways that establish the therapeutic alliance.

Note

1   This case is based on a clinical demonstration I did at the Milton H. Erickson 12th Conference in Phoenix, AZ on December 16, 2016. It was supposed to be a demonstration using chatting as brief therapy but ended up (as you will note) as a demonstration of guided imagery for psychotherapy, plus commentary on a variety of topics. Please note that Jennifer signed a waiver for this.

14 Case Study 8

Barbara and Stress and Hearing and a Husband

fog
mythifying the forest
only soft sounds

I believe that Barbara found out about me somehow online. She was willing to travel from three hours away, and she was interested in a hypnosis session since many other things she had tried had not worked. Barbara is 68 years old, retired, has two grown children, and a good marriage. She came to the session with her husband, Bob, who was there throughout. [I note here that Bob was quite skeptical about hypnosis, and also obviously quite protective of his wife.] Barbara mentioned that there was some stress in her life, that she had fibromyalgia, and that her main concern was hearing loss. She had been to the usual doctors like ENT specialists. She had also heard that hypnosis might help with various physical problems and might be of some use in increasing her understanding of what she heard.[1]

Barbara had also written to me (we communicated via email) that she thought that "my issue is most likely mind related." After some general conversation I decided that guided imagery would be the appropriate way to work with Barbara. Upon asking her what would work for her I found out: (1) prayer was relaxing and also paying attention to her breathing; (2) her safe haven was being near the ocean; and (3) that God would be her healing entity. I also asked her permission to hold her hand at some time during the hypnosis part. She and her husband were interested in some additional information about hypnosis, and I explained that it was basically focused attention. [Being protective, Bob asked her if she really wanted to do this. She was quite positive about going ahead.]

I am not going to repeat here the standard way of getting into such a session with paying attention to breathing and drifting off to the safe haven with some detail about being on a beach. When she was obviously in a trance state and relaxed and breathing easily, God visited her and with his healing power and knowledge and love and compassion was able to transfer to her ways of coping with and caring for herself with her hearing loss. [With her overly concerned husband being present I did not ask to hold her hand, but instead mentioned that via the sound vibrations in the air with the words I was using that somehow, also from me and through me, she would also be receiving healing messages and abilities and skills.]

Barbara left stating that she had got what she had come for, and her husband appeared convinced that hypnosis was okay and had helped her. I mentioned my sleep and relaxation CD and my guided imagery one, and upon their request sent them to her after the session. As is, usually the case with my clients, I have not heard back from Barbara. So, here is another example of using the guided imagery model to do a combination of psychotherapy and healing.

Note

1   I note here that hypnosis has helped in many physical concerns, pain control, allergies, stress, etc. In fact there is a whole volume of Milton Erickson's work using hypnosis for physical and physiological problems. One of his classical cases had to do with working with a man who had severe tinnitus. The main part of his intervention with this man was to tell a story of visiting a boiler factory with its incredibly loud noises when he was a student, and noting that the workers were actually able to communicate with each other through the din. After sleeping there overnight he found he could also understand the workers! As a personal note, I have had tinnitus for a long time but am only occasionally aware of this "shushing" background noise. I also generally am not aware of the loud (and incomprehensible to me!) music played in the weight room in which I work out.

15 Practical Matters

> across the morning
> half moon greets the sun
> the meadow wakens

15.1 Introduction

Life is both predictable and unpredictable. To live and survive in this world of chaos and uncertainty (perhaps, even survive!) we have learned how to plan for and guess at what seems at times to be random happenings. After they occur, our work is to cope realistically and practically with the existing realities. This chapter is devoted to summarizing and expanding on what I have written (Battino, 2001). Although the title of that book (*Coping. A Practical Guide for People with Life-Challenging Diseases and Their Caregivers*) appears on the surface to be narrowly focused, the coping skills described in it also extend to everyday life. For example, Chapter 5 on "Varieties of Coping" has 30 sections, only one of which deals directly with practical matters such as wills and powers of attorney. Since my book goes into quite a bit of detail on many subjects, I briefly describe here what I consider to be the most important of them here. Also, as my wife, Charlotte, and I get older (now 83 and 88), we have delved more into end-of-life issues, so I am devoting Appendix B to these matters.

15.2 Planning

A variety of practical matters will be covered here in brief sections. Advanced directives (such as living wills) are taken up in the end-of-life section. It is recommended that you consult a licensed attorney in your area for more specific and up-to-date guidance.

A. Financial and Legal Matters

I recall Ken, a member of a support group I was part of a long time ago, who showed up at a meeting with a thick three-ring binder. He had prostate cancer and the prognosis was not good. He told us that he did not want his family to be burdened by all of the practical and legal matters that would show up after he had died. That binder contained all of the information they would need to expeditiously take care of these matters. (I hasten to add here that no matter how carefully you prepare all of these things, there are some that will be missed, and also court and financial institutions do not respond rapidly.) Nevertheless, it behooves us to minimize the burdens of those we leave behind.

The main legal issues that need to be handled are wills and powers of attorney. A legally binding will gives directions about the disposition of all of your worldly goods after death. The more detail that is in your will, the better. You need to specify who will be the executor of your will. It can be more than one person, it can be an institution like a bank, and it can be a lawyer or a law firm. Whoever takes on the executor job needs to be someone you know and trust, and with whom you have consulted and also received their agreement in advance. Generally, this is a family member. Some executors are paid for this service. You can find forms for wills online, but it is best to use the services of a lawyer for preparing a will. Also, wills should be updated on a regular basis as your own and others' circumstances change. Wills need to be properly witnessed and notarized. It is prudent to have copies of your will deposited in your bank, and with your lawyer and children and trusted friends and the designated executor. Wills can be sealed or open. As many people get older down-sizing their possessions becomes important, and you may wish to actively do this while it easy for you. As older people who have had to down-size possessions, my wife and I have had the quite common experience of discovering that our children are not much interested in inheriting our family heirlooms or the items we cherish (and we thought that they would love to have!). Estate planning is important. In this regard, I recall visiting some old friends who had a large collection of art and artifacts and were just going to leave all of that stuff to their children to clear up. This is not recommended.

I have witnessed that many of my older friends and relatives become less able as they age to take care of their finances. Balancing a check book can be a problem for anyone! When my wife's mother had trouble doing this, my wife took over her mother's finances. That is, my mother-in-law gave her daughter power of attorney over all of her finances. This is a legal document and needs to be properly drawn up and witnessed. At the time of this writing my oldest brother was 99 years old and his three children shared his power of attorney; he did this even though he was still capable of doing much of this himself. (He has since died.) We all need to recognize when it is time to give up driving a car because our faculties have diminished, and also time to let others control our finances.

B. Planning Beyond Life

It is prudent to plan on what happens to your body after you die. You can make individual plans with a local funeral home and cemetery, and you can make plans via organizations you can join. For the former you can pay in advance or set aside funds for this purpose. The brother I mentioned above was president for over 25 years of the burial society of a Greek/Jewish group in the New York City area. A paid-up member of this group was guaranteed a burial plot in one of the cemeteries with which the society contracted. In Jewish tradition a dead person must be buried within 24 hours of death (if possible). Membership in this society also included the costs of the funeral service, although more expensive coffins could be purchased.

My wife and I belong to two memorial societies: the Funeral Consumers Alliance (FCA), which has branches in most states (if we happen to die more than 25 miles from where we now live); and the memorial society of our local Unitarian Fellowship. FCA has a single low membership fee, and organizes cremation for a negotiated low cost. The Unitarian group (of which I am an active member) has arranged for a reasonable fee for a local funeral home to pick up the body of the member who has died, and take them to a nearby crematorium for cremation.

In our area the Township runs the Glen Forest Natural Cemetery. Some people make the choice of a "natural" burial in which their body is covered in a shroud and then buried six feet down in the ground. The cost for natural burials can be significantly lower than other choices.

Although it is rare, some people (or their friends and relatives) arrange for a meeting of appreciation and recognition of their lives when they are still alive. This occurred for one of my close friends, and we all had a great time talking about him, telling stories, laughing together, and having a communal meal. In this way you can "be there" rather than assume a grand memorial service!

Where I live (Yellow Springs, OH) it has become a tradition that after a person dies that there will be a "celebration of life" community memorial service. Since my volunteer work is with people who have (or had) life-challenging diseases, I have experience in both organizing and facilitating such meetings.[1] Most of the time these celebration of life services are organized by family, but I have had the honor of arranging such services in advance with some of the people with whom I have spent time. You can write out those plans in advance, and you can also write your own obituary.

Life insurance and long-term care insurance are other considerations. Some people find that purchasing life insurance is a good deal financially in terms of planning for the future. Generally, it is economically better to obtain it when you are younger. It is better to obtain guidance in this from impartial sources other than insurance companies themselves. Long-term care insurance can be quite expensive, especially if you obtain it too late in life. My wife and I have long-term care insurance that we obtained over ten years ago. There are not many insurance companies that do this now. We basically purchased it and maintain it since we do not want to put a burden on our children if we need it, and it still appears to be an economically sound choice. Again, there are independent consumer groups and governmental agencies that can provide non-profit information.

15.3 Physical Health Related Coping Skills

In this section under various headings we consider coping skills related to physical health. Many of them are involved with hospitals and medical personnel. Again, this is an introduction to the subject.

A. How to Survive in a Hospital

The psychologist Lawrence LeShan (1990, pp. 80–100) has spent many years working with terminally ill patients in hospitals. See his full list for completeness. Here are some of his recommendations (some with citations and others paraphrased):

- Hospitals generally define a *good patient* as one who accepts their actions and statements uncritically and unquestionably. On the other hand, a *bad patient* is one who raises problems, asks questions to which they do not have answers, and does not accept hospital procedures as necessarily useful, wise, or intelligent.
- If at all possible, have a relative or friend with you who can serve as an advocate.
- Before you enter the hospital, there are certain facts you should have and certain questions you should ask. (1) Who is the physician who has the overall responsibility for your care? (2) What is the diagnosis, and how certain of it is your physician? (3) What is the usual course of the disease, both with and without therapy? (4) What are the side effects of the therapy? (5) What alternatives exist? ... Will the physician's course of action change depending on the results of the test? *If not, there is no reason to take it.* (pp. 88–89) [RB note: most of these questions can be asked of any physician.]
- When you are speaking to a physician about an illness, keep checking to make sure that you are hearing each other. [Do this check for any communication with health providers.]

- Control the number of people who will give you physical examinations.
- Have your physician write out for you all of the medications you are supposed to get, what each looks like, and at what times you should get them.
- Feel free to complain.
- You have the right to know the results of all of your tests and examinations.
- You can leave the hospital at any time.

B. Milstein's Comments and Coping Suggestions

Linda Milstein's book (1994, 2004) lists hundreds of practical suggestions for coping, especially for giving comfort for one who is ill. On Amazon.com I found just a few copies available and the following single review,

> I just finished reading this book and had to write to say that it was so helpful—it provided very realistic, 'easy', and important ideas of things to do for someone ill, either in the hospital or at home. I bought it because my 11 year old son is very ill and I feel so helpless—this book gave me ideas of both little AND big things I can do to help bring him comfort. It also talks about ways for the caregiver to take care of himself or herself which I found also very useful. Thank you for such a helpful and easy-to-read book!

Since what she writes is so useful, I am going to copy here from my book on coping (Battino, 2001) the items I singled out, and by her numbered suggestions. (I learned about this book a long time ago from one of the founders of Hospice of Dayton as she told me they referred many of the relatives and friends of their patients to this book.)

1 Show that you care by simply being there.
2 Make short, frequent visits that will not wear you or your loved one out.
3 If she is tired and weak, she may simply like to hear your voice, in person or over the phone, even if she doesn't feel like talking.
4 Help your loved one keep friendships going.
5 Be a friendly listener.
6 Be an honest friend … there is nothing you can say about your loved one's illness that she hasn't already thought of in private.
7 Listen unreservedly to your loved one's reports of her physical and medical changes and routines.
8 Listen tolerantly to your loved one's anger at old wounds, new hurts, life, the current situation. Listen uncritically to complaints, large and small, real and imagined.

9 Listen bravely to your loved one's fears, worries, and uncertainties. ... You cannot truly travel with your loved one on the road in this illness. But you can accompany this special person in facing her secret concerns.

10 Listen compassionately to your loved one's treatment plans (or plans to refuse treatment).

11 Praise your loved one for all of the good things in her life. Appreciate the positive: her good qualities, friendships, and happy experiences.

12 Forgive your loved one for past grievances.

13 Ultimately your loved one must die without you. Do not leave him first, emotionally, before he has a chance to leave you in reality.

14 Tolerate. Tolerate your loved one's anger without returning it. Tolerate your loved one's fear without succumbing to it.

15 Gather strength from your own good health. Take especially good care of your physical condition. Do not ignore little symptoms or neglect routine check-ups and medical and dental care. Do not compare your problems with your loved one's. Your first job is to keep well, so you can do all the other things you want to do.

Physical touch is the most important and immediate way to express your feelings for your loved one.

(p. 53) [Italics added since I believe this is extremely important.]

It's often easy to lose sight of the person behind the illness. Your loved one may be sick, perhaps quite seriously, but your relationship is with the person, not the illness.

(p. 69)

You cannot stop death, or avoid it, or defeat it, or take your loved one's place in it. You can, however, be alongside your loved one when she dies. Your presence is, and always was, the best comfort you can give.

(p. 99)

It can be comforting to talk about the hopes and plans that he is not able to fulfill himself, but would want others to continue in his absence. Anticipating the future together can make your loved one feel he has a share in it.

(p. 102)

Giving yourself some of the comfort and care you have given your loved one will help restore your capacity to give more in the future.

(p. 121)

Milstein also emphasizes the importance of *listening* and just *being there*.

C. Communicating with Medical Personnel

Perhaps the first thing to keep in mind is that you are the purchaser of medical services and that *they work for you*. When we get a new member of our support group (Charlie Brown) almost one of the first things we tell them is that if they are not satisfied with their doctor (or other medical personnel) that they can "fire" them and change them. Similarly, if you do not like the hospital or other medical facility you are in, you can ask to be transferred to another one. For example, Catholic Church affiliated health institutions have certain restrictions based on their religious beliefs (the right to have an abortion is one of them). Medical personnel typically refer to their clients as "patients," but you do not have to be patient! (On a personal note, I once had a dentist who specialized in root canal work who always had you in his dental chair exactly at the time of the appointment!)

You have the right to see and receive copies of all of your medical records. All of the medical and dental personnel my wife and I go to now automatically give us copies of their notes on our visits, as well as any tests that were performed. (Occasionally, these are mailed to us. Also, almost all health organizations have "portals" you can sign up with to get copies of your records and other information.) Hospitals also have to give you copies of all of the paperwork relating to both medical and financial information they have regarding your stay or visit there. For instance, the financial records for my several day stay in a hospital to get a knee replacement ran to almost 20 pages!

Many medical doctors now hand out printed information about their diagnoses and instructions for post treatment. If you do not get this automatically, ask for it. Also, pharmacies will give you printed information about any prescription drugs you purchase (again, you may have to ask for this). When I check out at my local pharmacy, I have to indicate in the financial card machine that I have been offered information relevant to a prescription.

Some doctors are quite formal and others are not. Since I am invariably older than my doctors, I ask them if it would be okay to be on a first name basis. I have yet to be refused, although one doctor asked me to not do so when other personnel were around!

When I know that a visit to a doctor will be an important one (about possible surgery or the results of tests for a major illness), I bring along an advocate who can take notes and maybe ask questions, and also a miniature solid state recording device. (These are readily available for prices below $50.) I always ask permission to record the session. Although a few of my doctors appeared to be reluctant to allow this, they all have. Most people (including me) go into a "zombie" like state or stasis when receiving a diagnosis and a prognosis related to a serious medical intervention or diagnosis. That is, we have an extremely limited memory of what the doctor told us. I have listened to these recordings afterwards, and even transcribed portions of them. You cannot comply or carry out the doctor's instructions unless you have some record of them! It is now over 30 years ago that Meichenbaum and Turk (1987) wrote about studies on *adherence* or *compliance*. Actually, compliance with doctor's instructions is very low. Although the treatment for diabetes mellitus is very well known and following the regimen is not burdensome, Meichenbaum and Turk found that compliance was less than fifty per cent.

A recent article in *HealthDay News* cites eight reasons associated with patients' intentional nonadherence to medications that were identified in a report published by the American Medical Association (AMA, Oct. 16, 2015). They note that data show about one-quarter of new prescriptions are never filled, and that about 50% of the time patients do not take their medication. According to the report, fear of potential side effects is one main reason for intentional nonadherence. In addition, cost may affect whether patients fill their prescriptions or ration their medication supply. Misunderstanding the need for medication, the nature of side effects, and the time taken to see results also affects nonadherence. Other factors that impact nonadherence include having too many medications, lack of symptoms, concerns about becoming dependent on medications, and depression. Mistrust of the doctor's motivations behind prescription of certain medications also influences nonadherence. It turns out that most nonadherence is intentional, that is, patients make a rational decision not to take their medicine based on their knowledge, experience, and beliefs. With respect to mistrust, patients may be suspicious of their doctor's motives for prescribing certain medications because of recent news coverage of marketing efforts by pharmaceutical companies influencing physician prescribing patterns.

Here is information from two more recent articles on compliance. Jin, et al. (2008), did a review from the perspective of patients on factors causing therapeutic non-compliance. They did a literature search (102 articles) of the Medline database from 1970 to 2005. They categorize factors related to compliance as being "hard" or "soft." "Hard" factors are said to be amenable to a certain extent by counseling and communication by healthcare providers. On the other hand, "soft" factors can be classified as psychosocial ones such as the patient's beliefs, and their attitude towards therapy and their motivation to therapy. They describe *adherence* as the ability and willingness to abide by a prescribed therapeutic regimen. Here are a number of observations made by Jin, et al., and cited (from the literature) in their paper:

- Generally speaking, it was estimated that the compliance rate of long-term therapy medication therapies was between 40% and 50%. The rate of compliance for short-term therapy was much higher at between 70% and 80%, while the compliance with lifestyle changes was the lowest at 20% and 30%.

- The rates of non-compliance with different types of treatment also differ greatly, e.g. (1) Estimates showed that almost 50% of the prescription drugs for the prevention of bronchial asthma were not taken as prescribed; (2) Patients' compliance with medication for hypertension was reported to vary between 50% and 70%; (3) Among adolescent outpatients with cancer, the rate of compliance with medication was reported to be 41%, while among teenagers with cancer it was higher at between 41% and 53%; (4) For the management of diabetes, the rate of compliance among patients to diet varied from 25% to 65%, and for insulin administration it was about 20%; and (5) More than 20 studies published in the last few years found that compliance with oral medication for type 2 diabetes mellitus ranged from 65% to 85%.
- Prescribing medication with a non-invasive route of administration (e.g., oral medication) and simple dosing regimens might motivate patients to be more compliant.
- Non-compliance is usually not a prevalent issue in acute illness or illness of short duration. In contrast, patients who are suffering from chronic diseases, particularly those with fluctuation or absence of symptoms (e.g., asthma and hypertension) are likely to be non-compliant.
- If the patient feels that the cost of therapy is a financial burden, the compliance with therapy will definitely be threatened.

The article by Czobor and Skolnick (2011) comments on the high failure rate of drugs in clinical trials in the abstract to their article:

The high failure rate of drugs in clinical trials, especially in the later stages of development, is a significant contributor to the costs and time associated with bringing new molecular entities to market. These costs, estimated to be in excess of $1.5 billion when capitalized over the ten to fifteen year required to develop a new entity, are one of the principal drivers responsible for the ongoing entrenchment of the pharmaceutical industry. Therapeutic areas such as psychiatry, now deemed very high risk, have been widely downsized, if not abandoned entirely, by the pharmaceutical industry. The extent to which patient noncompliance has marred clinical research has in some cases been underestimated, and one step to improving the design of clinical trials may lie in better attempts to analyze patent compliance during drug testing and clinical development.

This is an interesting and related approach to the compliance area.

D. Helplessness, Hopelessness, and Control

It may be that in their training many doctors were told to not give " false hope" to patients. They base their prognoses on the "hard" evidence of medical tests, their experience, and the outcomes of various studies related to that particular disease or collection of symptoms. The studies (if done properly) *all have error bars* associated with them. And, in modern times, studies are double-blind and involve placebos. So, skilled doctors, like any experienced professional, can make informed guesses about what is causing the disease and what treatments are likely to be helpful in a cure or mitigating its progress. (In a similar way we trust the "diagnoses" of an experienced car mechanic who listens to the engine, runs tests, and examines the car.) When someone gets a diagnosis of a life-challenging disease and the accompanying prognosis of possible treatments, and perhaps even life expectancy, they will almost all enter a fugue state, become hopeless, feel a sense of helplessness, and feel that they no longer have control over their life. This may be for a short or a long time. Any sense of hope, even a glimmer, can fire up the body's and mind's defense systems and energy to cope and to challenge. Thus, hope can really be a positive driving force in coping with the diagnosis and prognosis and illness.

One of the most inspiring and hopeful and practical books I have come across in this regard was written by Stephen H. Schneider (2005). The title and subtitle of the book are, *The Patient From Hell. How I worked with my doctors to get the best of modern medicine and HOW YOU CAN TOO.* Schneider, a climate scientist at Stanford and a MacArthur fellow, brought skills rooted in the uncertainties in his own field to bear on the treatments he received for mantle cell lymphoma, a rare condition for which treatments were relatively new. With his wife, Terry, also a scientist, he learned as much as possible about the protocol he had been assigned, and read up on his oncologist. He gives a detailed account of the painful and otherwise unpleasant side effects of the chemotherapy and other treatments. From the beginning Schneider researched probabilities and outcomes and sought to modify decisions made by his physicians. His scientific language can be daunting, but patients will relate to his arguments for the importance of patient advocates, individualization of treatments, and the negative role bottom-line accounting plays in medical judgments made by HMOs. The significant message here for me is how Schneider took his diagnosis and *prognosis as a challenge* to his inquiring scientific mind, and how he was actually able to convince his oncologist to use treatments that actually prolonged his life beyond the initial prognosis.

It is normalizing to know that almost everyone who gets the diagnosis of a life-challenging disease and the accompanying prognosis is to feel depressed, hopeless, helpless, and out of control. Knowing this lets the person move on.

I have even had a number of people I know tell me that they consider that the diagnosis of cancer has been a "gift." On the surface this seems strange.

But, then they go on to explain that this "gift" has forced upon them the knowledge that their life is really finite, and that they now have the job of figuring out what is really important in their lives, and how to live that way. That is, most of us (even those quite old) do not have the opportunity to consciously work on planning the rest of their life in terms of what they can now do. Will they write out a "bucket list" of what they are going to do before they kick that bucket? Is *now* the time to do which of "all those things" that they were going to do? In a way, this becomes the relief of having the "permission" to ignore some things and really work at others. Paradoxical, yes, and freeing up also.

E. Hammerschlag's Recommendations and Laughter

My friend Carl Hammerschlag (1988, 1993) has listed many recommendations on his web site (www.healingdoc.com). Here are a few of them:

- Be positive and celebrate life.
- Appreciate your own uniqueness and self-worth.
- Recognize that adversity is part of life and deal with it in a positive way.
- Take action. Make choices. Take care of your unfinished business.
- Heal your spirit. Deal with fear. Look at your life differently.
- Live in the present. Listen to your heart.
- Be consistent in thought, word, and deed.
- Let go of anger. Look to serve others.
- Become a visionary. Love others and seek love in return.
- Believe and have faith. Pray.

Many of the waiting rooms I have been in had old copies of the *Reader's Digest* with which I whiled away the time being "patient." I invariably looked at the word definition game and also "Laughter-the Best Medicine." And, it is. A good "belly laugh" from a joke or a cartoon or pun or a sight gag can bring tears to your eyes and a stitch in your side. Being able to laugh at yourself, in particular, is excellent medicine, "How could I have done that?" You just know that when people are laughing together that they are having fun and enjoying life and are free from the worries that seem to crop up in our lives. The most remarkable story I know about the benefits of laughter are when Norman Cousins (1979) literally used laughter to cure himself of ankylosing spondylitis, rheumatoid arthritis of the spine where the connective tissue progressively disintegrates with no known cause or cure. This was done with medical advice. Laughter, of course, is not a guaranteed cure, yet it can ease awkward and difficult situations. You might even say, if what you are doing isn't FUN, what is it? Also, since you cannot be physiologically panicked and relaxed at the same time, which one will you choose?

F. Maintaining Mental and Physical Health

Counseling and psychotherapy can help in many ways. People get stuck in various patterns of behavior and with various habits, and a professional therapist can help in those circumstances. They specialize in guiding you to be able to make more choices in your life and to break out of restrictive patterns. I mentioned earlier that almost everyone who gets a diagnosis of a life-challenging disease goes through being depressed for some time. It is useful to know that this is a common reaction, and that help is available from individual therapists and from support groups. Many studies have shown that psychotherapy helps most of the people who use it. (There are also studies that show that many people get through these difficult times on their own!) Medical doctors can refer you to a relevant support group. Since medical doctors have a tendency to refer patients to psychiatrists, if you wish to see a counselor or psychotherapist or social worker, then you need to get a referral from someone in those fields. There are many publicly funded mental health agencies. For older people most senior centers and county councils on aging can provide referrals. Also, personal referrals from friends or family members who have been in therapy are good. If you are a member of a religious group, then the minister usually can provide referrals or help himself or herself.

My simple model of psychotherapy is that when a person gets stuck that they have only one response or one emotional response to a given stimulus or situation. A good therapist guides you into having more appropriate responses and emotional reactions. That is, you then have more choices in your life. The last time I looked there were well over 600 "named" psychotherapies. In competent hands they probably all have worked well with many clients. In my own practice I work as a very brief therapist, rarely seeing a client more than one time. This is called "single-session therapy" or SST. Studies of SST therapists show that the particular approach that they use is not a significant factor.

For many people, religion provides comfort and help in difficult times. Prayer can be particularly helpful. There is even some evidence that prayer can help in healing both mental and physical difficulties.

There are some writing things you can do that often help. One of them is keeping a journal or a diary. This practice was common many years ago, yet it can be quite helpful. It may be done for specific purposes, but most often a diary or journal is kept as a personal log of feelings, ideas, observations, and activities. In terms of mental health, there may be things that you feel uncomfortable sharing with a spouse or a close friend, yet you can write about it for your own comfort or release. It is a place to keep personal secrets and feelings.

G. Work Books and Distance Writing

Another way of writing that has been designed for mental health is called structured writing or distance writing or programmed writing. This is different than keeping a journal or a diary in that you are guided by a series of questions focused on a particular concern or difficulty. For example, Pennebaker (1997, pp. 20–25, 73–88) has written about structured writing for grieving.[2] In my book on coping (Battino, 2001) I give three complete workbooks like this for people who have cancer or other life-challenging disease, for grievers, and for caregivers. To give you a better sense of what these workbooks are like, I copy here the first group of questions for each of them. (Please note that there may be as many as 20 questions in these workbooks.)

Workbook for People who Have Cancer or other Life-Challenging Disease

1   Use the following space to respond to these three related questions. You may not be able to answer them with any certainty—in that case, you may have a guess or a theory about how to answer these questions. (a) Why is this happening to me (vs. someone else)? (b) Why is this happening to me at this particular time of my life? (c) Why do I have this particular kind of cancer or disease?

2   Do you know, or do you have a theory, or can you guess as to why at this particular time you are doing better, or worse, or staying the same?

3   What ways of taking care of yourself are you waiting to explore? (These can be things like: second or third opinions, more research on available medical treatments, alternative or complementary treatments, support groups, support networks, or personal things like counseling/psychotherapy.)

Workbook for Grievers

1   Write in detail about the good ties you have had with the person whose loss you are grieving.

2   Write about losses that you shared and experienced together.

3   What special personal characteristics will see you through this time?

4   What are your special strengths?

5   What ways of taking care of yourself are you willing to explore at this time? How will you overcome things that are in the way of you taking care of yourself?

6   What is different about the times you when you are able to function normally? How can you extend those times?

Workbook for Caregivers

1   The following three questions are related. You may not be able to answer them with certainty—in that case, you may have a guess or a theory about how to answer these questions. (a) Why is this happening to the person I love (vs. someone else)? (b) Why is this happening to her/him at this particular time? (c) Why does he/she have this particular disease (vs. a different one)?

2   Do you know or do you have a theory, or can you guess why he/she is doing better, worse, or staying the same at this time?

3   Write in detail about the good times you have had with the person for whom you are caring.

4   Write about the special memories or experiences the two of you have shared.

5   Write about losses that you have shared and experienced together.

6   What special characteristics will see you through this time?

7   What are your special strengths?

I trust that the above examples give you some idea as to how these "workbooks" with their organized series of questions can help a person through a difficult time by writing about it.

Support groups where there is an agreement by all participants to keep what is said there in strict confidentiality are places where you can share your innermost thoughts and emotions and fears, know that you are being heard, and finding an inner release and comfort from being open. In the support group I facilitated this is a central part of providing support to the members.

There are many alternative and complementary methods that have been promulgated and advertised for healing diseases. It is probable that all of them have helped someone, but the scientific evidence is rarely there, and one needs to be cautious. I have heard Bernie Siegel say that it if you want to try one of these approaches, do it, but also always do it in conjunction with medical guidance and advice. I just note in passing here the TV commercials for all sorts of prescription drugs for seemingly endless diseases: however, if you *listen* to all of the potential side effects of taking those drugs, I find it hard to believe that anyone would really consult their doctor about trying them! (Oddly, the only two countries in the world that permit such advertising are America and New Zealand.)

Physical exercise is a super way to stay in good health. There are a great many regimens. Walking is an easy exercise and available to all of us. So, walk every day, and slowly increase the length of the walk, its speed, and duration (within your capacity). It turns out that we get the most benefit from exercises that use the big muscles in the legs. One thing I do is "interval training" on my home exercise bike. I do this almost every day and it takes 12 minutes in the following pattern: pedal easily for one minute, cycle fast for 20 seconds, cycle slowly for 100 seconds, repeat this pattern five times, and then slow down gradually for the last two minutes. From what I have read this is better than cycling for 12 minutes at a steady rate. Weight training is also quite good, but it is not aerobic. An interesting phenomenon is that when you do any exercise in which the bones are compressed (put under some stress) that this signals the body to strengthen *all* of the bones in your body. On the other hand, doing curls, leg or other lifts, etc., seems to strengthen just the muscles being used. So, it is important to do some weight-bearing exercises in your regimen. It is also recommended that when you do weight-bearing exercises that you exercise a given muscle or set of muscles *every other day* to give the muscles a chance to react. Jogging and cycling and stepping machines, etc., are all good. When you do aerobic exercises, the general recommendation is that you do them at such a rate that you could converse with someone who is doing it along with you. (Athletes, of course, push these limits.) There is some evidence that "fidgeting," that is, moving a lot during your day (rather than sitting in one position for a long time) is beneficial. So, get up and move around periodically. One other interesting phenomenon has to do with people who are ill and have to stay in bed in a hospital (or other setting). Muscles tend to atrophy in their strength more rapidly than most people think with even short bed rests of two or three days. So, if at all possible, in such circumstances get up and move around. A while back I was in hospital for three days and was tethered to an IV pole on casters—I made it a point to get up and walk around the ward regularly with my pole.

H. Diets

It is essential to pay attention to what you eat. There are, of course, endless diets promulgated to keep you healthy. In my coping book (Battino, 2001), my friend H. Ira Fritz, Ph.D., wrote the chapter entitled "Nutrition and Life-Challenging Diseases." He was the professor of nutrition at my university for many years. Also, he was my source for nutrition information whenever I had any questions. So, in this section I am going to briefly describe and give references to the three nutritional approaches in which he had the most confidence. They are:

1 U. S. Department of Agriculture's Food Pyramid—Their basic recommendation is to eat three to five servings of vegetables and two to four servings of fruit each day. Their website is: www.cnpp.usda.gov/FGP. In that site you can download the 17-page *Food Guide Pyramid Booklet*, which will give you much useful detailed information. Also, see their Food and Nutrition Information Center for many additional resources.

2 Dean Ornish (M.D.) is an oncologist who has designed an intervention program for the reversal of heart disease. It is basically a low-fat vegetarian diet, an exercise program emphasizing walking, programmed relaxation, and group interaction and support. He asserts that the combination of all of parts of the program is what makes it effective. His book (Ornish, 1991) contains details on his program.

3 The Traditional Healthy Mediterranean Diet Pyramid (Gifford, 1998) lays out nine levels of nutrition, with the lower levels indicating daily intake, and the upper levels showing foods that should be eaten only a few times per week or a few times per month. For example, the following are daily foods: breads, pasta, rice, couscous, polenta, other grains, potatoes, fruits, legumes, and other nuts, vegetables, olive oil in variable amounts, cheese, and yogurt; the following are for a few times each week: fish, poultry, eggs, and sweets; red meat is recommended for a few times a month or somewhat more in small amounts.

The bottom line on nutrition is just being sensible in what and how much you eat.

I. Recordings and Autobiographies

I started a long time ago making audio recordings of some of the people in the original Charlie Brown support group. Recall that these were people who had life-challenging diseases or were caregivers. Those with serious ailments all had prognoses of a shortened life. A psychologist named Janette Rainwater (1979) has written about her experience with geriatric clients with respect to the importance in telling their life stories. There are two relevant chapters in her book ("On Keeping a Journal," and "The Use of Autobiography"), and her book is still available. The significance here is that in telling (and retelling) the stories of your life that there is a *self-validation* that is both comforting and reassuring not only for older people, but for anyone. And, this is particularly true when facing a fore-shortened life. Indeed, the very act of telling or writing about your life history, activities, achievements (and even failures) will bring your life into perspective, root it in history, and *give it value and meaning*. I highlighted the last phrase since we are not always aware of or appreciative of what *we* have done in our lives. There are lives we have touched and people who have touched ours. There are places we have traveled to that were special, and there were forgotten "magic" moments that existed in the specialness of "ordinary" living. In this regard I remember the poignant scene in Thornton Wilder's "Our Town" where Emily (after death) returns to Grover's Corners and recalls the magic of everyday growing up there. Writing your autobiography or your memoirs is one way to do this.[3]

I started making voice recordings in the era before inexpensive videotaping. The early tape recordings were of members of the support group before

I realized that it made sense to also do this for older family members (I have recordings of my older sister and my father), and older friends. The video tapes are generally two hours long. I lead them through their life starting with when and where they were born, information about their parents, where they grew up, how and where their parents met, where they lived and their occupations. Then it is asking them about their earliest memories and about any siblings. What was their life like when they were a child, a pre-teen, a teen, and a young adult? What was their social life along the way? How did they meet and fall in love with their spouse? When interviewing a husband and wife, elicit information separately up to the time of their marriage. And here are a bunch more questions to guide you if you do the interviewing: What was their early married life together like? What about occupations and avocations? If they have children, relate some strong and good memories about the children growing up and moving on. How much did they travel, and any good memories about places they visited? Are there grandchildren—and some comments and thoughts about them? Sons or daughters-in-law? Now, looking back, do they have any special advice or guidance for children and grandchildren? The ending is simply, "Anything else you would like to say?" Finally, you thank them for the privilege of learning about their life. The interview has the essence of gathering information as if you were going to be their biographer.

J. Some Final Comments

We have almost all been brought up with the caution that it is better to give than receive, and better to offer than to ask. Yet, one of the gifts that you can give someone is the opportunity for them to give something *to you*. When you need help (at any time of your life) remember that asking for help is giving others the chance to be a giver. Doing this can be hard.

A related idea is that there are times when it is important and useful to be selfish, as in taking care of yourself so you can take care of others or simply because you realistically need to do that. This may even be considered to be part of that advice that the best revenge is living well. Another connection is that of keeping or taking control over your life rather than bowing to other's wishes. This is related to Rabbi Hillel's question of, "If I am not for myself, who will be?"

Notes

1 In fact, I have prepared a "checklist" for this purpose. It is available upon request.
2 You can find more information about programmed writing in L'Abate and Cox (1992).
3 In this regard I have thoroughly enjoyed reading the four-part memoir of an old friend who grew up in Scotland. He has an extraordinary memory for his childhood and youth. There were many surprises for me since we met much later in our lives.

16 Case Study 9

Laura and Breaking Away

to a baby's hand
the world is something to grasp
its life is touching

I mentioned the "Yenta Syndrome" earlier and that is certainly something I have to be aware of since I live and work in a small town (ca. 4000), have had many local residents as clients, and run into them frequently. Occasionally, my wife knows who these people are, but never knows how many times I may have seen them or for what. Also, interestingly, it may actually be several decades since the last session. They know, of course, that I do not talk about them, and that if I do write up a case study like this one I mask their identity and even change what they came to see me about to something sufficiently parallel that there are no hints as to their identity. In addition, I am careful about asking permission to write up a case where appropriate. Laura is one of these clients.

She is in her late thirties and unmarried although she has had more than one long-term partner. I saw her twice with about 15 months in between. Laura had recurring "low" periods, and she also wanted some help with what she called "bad" habits. At the first session she indicated that her (current) relationship was going well, but they had gotten into some "bad" habits like smoking too much. There was also some anxiety about death,[1] but we did not get into that. Since it seemed that stopping smoking would be the entree to resolving a bunch of difficulties, we started with that.

The Narrative Therapy technique of externalization seemed to be the best choice of working with a habit that was out of control and driven by a compelling internal force of some kind. I posed this idea to Laura, and she decided to call her internal controlling smoking "imp" Red. So, the procedure then was to "exorcize" Red during a hypnosis session via the power of a healer who could do this. Laura easily went into a trance state by paying attention to her breathing. The healer came closer to her and was able to easily enter her body, locate Red, extract him (Red seemed to be male) and send him off into space to burn up in the sun to never be able to trouble her again. [Please note that I had earlier established that there were times when Laura could resist Red and be in control of her habit. This showed her that she did, indeed, have some control over her behavior.]

At this point I felt that Laura needed some additional internal strength to really feel in charge herself in these matters. [I had earlier asked her if it would be okay to hold her hand and she said "Yes."] I was aware that having known her for some time that she trusted me and had confidence in me. That is, I was someone she could rely on, and I felt at this time that a physical bonding was important. So, I reached out and we ended up holding both hands. Continuing with hypnotic language and intonation I said things like,

> Somehow, from me and through me, the removal of Red via the Healer was being reinforced and strengthened and made permanent. You can feel and sense this, can you not? There are some solid and concrete places in you now that will be there with you as you move forward, easily and simply, knowing ... now ... that Red is forever gone from your life, and you will be free of him at last ... free at last. And you will be able to remember and recall and store within you everything that you have learned, and all of the changes that have already occurred, will you not? Yes. And Yes. Thank you for your attention and trust and confidence. And, when you are ready, you can take a deep breath or two, stretch a bit, and open your eyes. Thank you.

[This ending is my (almost) standard way of closing a hypnosis session. Interestingly, during the last part of this session Laura cried a lot. I did not ask about this for some things are private, are they not? Also, for someone I knew this well, we did hug before she left.]

As I indicated above Laura returned for a second session about 15 months later, and with a different agenda. The relationship with her long-term partner was not working any more, she had new personal goals, and it was time for her to move on. My job, then, was to facilitate this course of change in her life. She initially told me that she was going to break with him in about six months at a special date in her life. Since she had made the decision to leave it was odd that she would put it off for so long. Our relationship was such that I function as an older wise relative to whom she could come to for guidance and advice and protection. In the last role it made no sense to me for Laura to stay in the relationship so long (before saying "so long!") and I decided to be *directive* in the sense of encouraging her to leave as soon as she could make the arrangements for another place to live. [Therapists are usually cautious about forcefully telling clients what to do in a given situation. Yet, there are times when the most important thing you can do for a client is to be open and direct and effectively say "You are nuts if you continue to act in this way and do not change immediately." I felt this way about Laura's current situation and went about it by first quoting Rabbi Hillel's three questions,[2] and then doing a guided imagery (GI) session to provide Laura with the necessary support and strength to make an immediate decision. Details on the GI session follow.]

For the GI session her choices were: (1) method of relaxing was paying attention to breathing; (2) safe haven was sunshine, beaches and forests; and (3) the healing modality was a healer, herbs like thyme, sunshine, and warm and kind spirits. In my usual way in a guided imagery session I incorporated all of these elements. In the healing modality portion I emphasized that her competence and strength and ability to act were all enhanced so that she could easily go forward with leaving, and cope with all aspects of what that entailed, especially her partner's anticipated reactions. We talked about the practicalities involved in leaving and moving into a new space and came up with many useful ideas, which she indicated she would explore and act upon. There was certainly much decisiveness in her at the end. To help herself in being sure about going ahead and to "protect" her she chose one of the small polished "anchor" stones (I have in a jar) to take with her. Laura is one of the few clients I get direct feedback from, and this was in an email from her, which I quote here, "I just wanted to say thank you for meeting with me a few weeks ago. About a week later, I left and have not been back since. It's been a few wild weeks, but an incredible time as well. I'm thankful to be in transition now." [It's always nice to get such feedback!]

Notes

1   I am going to get into this important issue here by quoting a description of I. D. Yalom's book (2009) entitled *Staring at the Sun: Overcoming the Terror of Death*, which I highly recommend as it concerns an issue that underlies many other things that clients present. The following is taken from his book, "Written in Irvin Yalom's inimitable story-telling style, *Staring at the Sun* is a profoundly encouraging approach to the universal issue of mortality. In this magisterial opus, capping a lifetime of work and personal experience, Dr. Yalom helps us recognize that the fear of death is at the heart of much of our anxiety. Such recognition is often catalyzed by an 'awakening experience'—a dream, or loss (the death of a loved one, divorce, loss of a job or home), illness, trauma, or aging. Once we confront our own mortality, Dr. Yalom writes, we are inspired to rearrange our priorities, communicate more deeply with those we love, appreciate more keenly the beauty of life, and increase our willingness to take the risks necessary for personal fulfillment."

I also recommend his related book (Yalom, 2017) entitled *Becoming Myself. A Psychiatrist's Memoir.*

2   About 2100 years ago Rabbi Hillel in his old age was asked to share his wisdom. He did so with the following three questions: (1) If I am not for myself, who will be? (2) If I am only for myself, what am I? (3) If not now, when? All three questions applied to Laura's current situation, and we discussed them with that in mind. They connected with her.

17 Case Study 10

George and Smoking

taught with tension
thunderclouds
lightning the night

I have worked with a number of teenagers over the years. George was sent to me by his father, someone I knew in our village, to help him stop smoking cigarettes and pot and to be more in charge of his life. He has a younger sister, and is into music at the high school. He told me that he had been smoking for a few years, and stopped for one week by vaping. Nicotine apparently calms him for a while and seems to act almost like a tranquilizer. The calming effect does not last, and he was apparently really interested in getting control of this part of his life.

Once again, I thought that the guided imagery format would be helpful. Paying attention to breathing was the opening. There were a number of places that George mentioned would be safe havens and places where he relaxed: a special place in the local forest preserve, walking in one place in town, one spot in his house, and a secluded woods area with lots of leaves on the ground. His healers were two people in the high school: a counselor named Willard and a music director named Fred. All of these elements were incorporated into a hypnosis/guided imagery session, which I have reconstructed as an illustration of this kind of work:

George, find a way of being comfortable in that arm chair, and then close your eyes if that is okay to do. Thank you. And, now, just pay attention to your breathing, noticing each breath as it comes in and goes out. Normally, easily, naturally. Just one breath at a time. One heartbeat at a time. And, with each inhale chest and belly softly rising. Then with each exhale all of those muscles just relaxing. You can even sense that each inhale is a kind of strengthening and calming one, while each exhale is a kind of clearing and freeing one. That's right, just one breath at a time. Occasionally, a stray thought may wander through, notice it, thank it for being there, and go back to this breath, and the next one.

And, now, within your mind you can just drift off to your special place in the woods, the calm and quiet and soft odors of the pine forest. Enjoy being there, perhaps sitting on one of the dead logs. The softness of the carpet of pine needles is all around, and high above a gentle breeze is blowing through the tree tops. While you continue to breathe in the peace of the pine forest, something interesting is happening. Somewhere near you, you sense the presence of Willard and Fred. And Willard comes close enough to perhaps even sit nearby. Somehow, his presence, the very air that you are both breathing, whatever he is saying or not saying is reassuring and calming. And, somehow, his voice, his words, and his presence are able in some interesting way to strengthen your sense of yourself, strengthen somewhere within your mind and body the knowledge, the conviction, the reality that from this time onward you will be able to stop smoking in a surprisingly easy way. There is part of you that resists this, and another part of you that is getting stronger and stronger with Willard's presence and words, so that deep within you— almost as if a switch were thrown—your no and knowing no that, yes, yes, I can, I will, I don't need that stuff any more. Wow. Wow. What a remarkable ... And, you thank Willard within your mind now, and perhaps you both smile and even grin. Yes, okay. And, Willard quietly moves away, leaving you with that inner sense of "Yes, I have. Yes, I am."

Fred now comes quietly towards you. I don't know whether he, too, sits on the log or is just nearby, perhaps surrounded by that aura of music that you can almost hear, can you not? And, you know that Fred has long been aware of your musical skills, ability, and ear. Somewhere, inside, you have come to know that you are a good musician, and in playing your instrument there is a sense of being, of well-being, of I can, and I have. There is between you and Fred something you note, notes perhaps, the very vibrations of music well-played. And you know, those vibrations, those notes within you have already helped strengthen your sense of self, your ability from this time on to take care of yourself without vapor and smoke. After all, vapor and smoke are ephemeral and vanish into the air, but those musical vibrations and frequencies resonate within, do they not? And, you and Fred look at each other, perhaps each thanking each other, and then Fred slowly withdraws.

Continuing to breathe softly, smoothly, easily. One breath, perhaps one note, at a time. And, George, you know that your mind will remember and recall what you have experienced here this afternoon. This may occur in the pine forest on another visit or in another of your special places. Change, George, can be almost instantaneous. And, I wonder ...

I want to thank you, George, for your trust and your attention, and when you are ready just take a deep breath or two, perhaps blink your eyes and stretch, and just come back to this room here and now. Thank you.

There was a look of calm and peace in George at this time, and perhaps also a bit of puzzle. I offered him my jar of small polished stones and suggested he take one to help him remember what had happened here this afternoon. He took one and we shook hands goodbye.

This session occurred over one year ago, and I do not know how much this changed George's life. All I know is that at the end of the session he appeared to have received what he wanted. (I also again note that the guided imagery model can be quite useful as a therapeutic change agent.)

18 Case Study 11

Peter and His PA

the musical note
softly vibrates air
moving chords with it

Peter was not having trouble with his father, he was having trouble with and was concerned about his Performance Anxiety (PA). Peter plays a brass wind instrument and has been doing so since he was ten or so. He is good enough to play in local brass and orchestral groups, but rarely plays solos. This PA was part of his life for a long time, and he told me that it is partly due to the high expectations his parents had for him. (Such expectations by parents are not unusual, and occasionally they do interfere with their children's life patterns.) Sometimes this becomes part of a "witch" message resulting in negative self-talk that hovers around in the back of the mind. The background here is that Peter (a man in his early seventies) came to see me since in two months he would be playing a solo as part of a community concert. The piece is a challenging one to learn and perform, and at this time he had much anxiety about it.

Since this had to do with self-image, I mentioned that I had doubts for a long time as to how good a chemistry professor I was. That is, I have felt for a long time that I was a bit of a hoax in the field[1] since I was certain that most of my colleagues were smarter in the subject than I was, and much better informed. I told him how surprised I was many years ago, when I was teaching in Chicago, to overhear one of my chemistry colleagues tell another one how much he admired me. I could not believe my ears. What was he thinking? What had I done to deserve that comment? Now, much later in life, I have much evidence in the popularity of my chemistry publications that I do have a good reputation in the field. I told Peter that those old messages are sometimes difficult to believe—*even in the face of evidence to the contrary*. He appeared to resonate with this comment by nodding and smiling.

I am one of those people who has a "tin ear" with respect to music. I then told a story to Peter about my encounter with music as a metaphor for finding fulfillment for the dreams and hopes we had about ourselves when we were young, and continue to exist in us throughout our lives. So, I told Peter that there was no one I knew in my family or community who did anything musical. My wife and our two sons have been involved with music their entire lives. So, in my mid-forties I decided to take up piano. I had a wonderful piano teacher who, however, made the mistake of not starting me out with ear training, i.e., being able to distinguish different notes. After five years of lessons and practice, I gave up the piano since I realized that I would never get much beyond playing "Three Blind Mice." On the other hand, I do have a big voice (which has come in handy in using hypnosis), so I decided that I would pursue my youthful dream of singing opera. I took voice lessons with a wonderfully patient and encouraging teacher for three years. By the end of that time I could actually sing a Mozart aria (from the "Marriage of Figaro"). The "but" here is that I could only sing this with a taped piano accompaniment of an opera singer. That is, I could match what he was doing. I ended my voice lessons soon after singing scales while my teacher played them on the piano, but did not recognize that I was off an entire octave! I told this story to Peter to indicate that one can realize a dream in different ways than being the "best" in any area.[2] This did connect with Peter.

At this point I decided that it made sense to use David Cheek's idiodynamic finger signaling approach to go back in time, and guide Peter into giving up his PA as no longer being necessary or applicable in his life. I suggested that via a series of questions, which his fingers would answer, that we would be able to resolve his concerns. So, I designated his forefinger as the "Yes" one, his middle finger as the "No" one, and his thumb as the "I am not ready to answer now" one. We rehearsed his responses via a series of standard Yes and No questions, and his thumb with "I have some questions about your sex life." (Peter closed his eyes for this part of the session, and was in a light trance.) After establishing when the PA started in his life via a series of questions as to when it had started, I used the Cheek question of, "Now that you are some 60 years older, and have been successfully in one of the helping professions for many years, would it be okay to just give up that unnecessary performance anxiety?" [I had already established that he was a competent musician, and was going to take lessons and guidance from a professional to be able to perform his solos well.] Perhaps to his surprise, his "Yes" finger immediately responded. I acknowledged that movement, and then went on to establish an anchor (of his choice) that he could use at the concert. [I generally suggest natural public movements like rubbing fingers together, making a gentle fist, or touching one's ear or nose or hair.] Peter chose rubbing fingers. I had him rehearse several times doing this while he thought about being at the performance. [This rehearsal when thinking about a future behavior is a wonderful anchor, and needs to be done several times.]

Before ending the session I felt that it would be useful to add one more reinforcement. To this end (Peter was still in a light trance) I did a Narrative

Therapy[3] related approach of a kind of "exorcism." I said to Peter: We can do one more thing now to reinforce these changes. [Implies that changes have *already* occurred.] There is a way to completely get rid of that big "A," no, let us call it the little "a." I do not know where little "a" is within you. Just imagine and feel now that it is dribbling out through your fingers, or perhaps through your feet and into the floor and all the way down to Earth's molten core, or even up through the top of your head and all the way out to the sun burning up and vanishing there. Just, little "a" completely vanishing from your body and your mind and your life. Yes. [Peter was smiling throughout this segment.]

And, Peter, I want to thank you for your trust and your confidence and your attention. Just take a deep breath or two, blink your eyes, and stretching a little, come on back to this room, here and now. Thank you.

At this point Peter appeared to be quite calm and relaxed. I asked if there was anything else he wanted to talk about. He said, "No." Then he started talking about his anxiety as if it were still there (perhaps in the background). He said things like, "You know I still feel a bit anxious about playing" and "I seem to still feel some anxiety." I interrupted this litany of talking about the old PA, and asked him to say, "The anxiety I *used to have*" several times in different ways. [He looked quite relieved after doing this.]

Just one more thing before you leave. You have noticed this jar of polished stones on the table. Please reach in and take one to remind you and be with you of all that has happened here this afternoon. [He did so, and told me he would keep it with him.]

Commentary 1

You will notice that the session began with us just having a chat, and me telling a personal story. I thought it was important to establish several things. One was the difficulty we often have about giving up old opinions and beliefs about ourselves (despite evidence to the contrary). Another was to share with Peter my experiences with music, and how I achieved success in an alternate (but acceptable to me) manner. [In a sense I was a fellow sufferer in both of these ways. Peter could enjoy playing his instrument without having to be the "best."]

The Cheek idiodynamic finger approach can be used in this simple way in just getting rid of old behaviors and beliefs. I decided to use this method since it was different, perhaps even novel, and fast, and I expected unknown to Peter. I also wanted to use it to go directly to his earliest experiences with PA to remove that hindrance at the root, so to speak. Clients generally have not thought that their life experiences up to their present life have really taught them that they *no longer need* those old inhibiting messages and ways of reacting, and can simply give them up. The power of this method is that, in effect, you are just giving your client *permission* to change!

I have found in working with PA clients that it is important to provide them with anchors (ordinary body movements) that remind them that they are okay and comfortable now in being a presenter. As I indicated above, it is important to *rehearse* the use of this anchor while envisioning the future activity. It seemed to me that Peter also needed to have little "a" completely removed from his system, so we did that via that little exorcism.

The addition of the Gestalt Therapy style[4] of statement about the little "a" he *used to have* brought a smile with some astonishment to his face. And, of course, there was that final anchor in Peter selecting a stone to keep with him as a reminder. Perhaps any one of the approaches I described above may have worked alone—in this case certainly more was better!

The evidence for the success of this session would, of course, be Peter's solos in the upcoming concert. However, that concert is two months away from this writing. (Subsequently, I ran into Peter in town and he told me that the concert and his solos went well.)

Commentary 2

Peter referred a colleague of his to me who has a similar PA. I will call her Anabel. There were only two things I did with Anabel in our session, and since only one was similar to the work I did with Peter, I think that it is worthwhile to briefly describe that session.

One of the things I have done in the past with PA clients (and I believe many other therapists do something similar) is to get them to think about situations where they feel good about themselves and are acting competently. I have them *anchor* that competence and state in a simple normal and everyday gesture. For Anabel this was touching an ear. I suggested that she close her eyes and think about the upcoming event. Then, at some appropriate time before the event started, she was to touch her ear. I asked her as a rehearsal to repeat this two more times. She "returned" to the room with a smile, which indicated to me that this little exercise worked. Anabel told me that she had tried visualization to prepare for performances and it helped a bit. There was a fear of failure. I recalled Bernie Siegel's comment about this and told her, "You know there is no such thing as failure, there are only different kinds of feedback." This reframing made sense to her.

I decided that it would be useful to adapt the guided imagery approach as an extra way to change her feelings about performing. She was comfortable with breathing as a way to relax, and her "safe haven" was being on a farm at haying time. When I asked what sort of healing and helping modality she would select I suggested several ways that music could be used. What would it be like if she heard an orchestral piece or quartet where her instrument was played as a solo? She thought about that and surprised me by saying that she would like to hear Frank Sinatra sing one of his songs. So, we did that with incorporating his voice as somehow moving throughout her entire body and changing it cell by cell, organ by organ, and nerve by nerve so that she would be completely at ease and comfortable when performing. The kind of "fog" that had interfered with performance before was totally dissipated and removed by Sinatra's voice!

I ended in my usual way of reinforcing the changes and indicating that she could re-experience what had gone on in this session whenever she needed to. When roused, Anabel appeared to be both relaxed and a bit surprised. I then asked her to choose a solid reminder from my jar of smooth small polished stones. This small gift at the end of a session continues to be received by her and other clients as both a surprise and a "solid" reassurance that the session has been helpful.

Notes

1   An interesting book about the "imposter phenomenon" is *The Impostor Phenomenon: Overcoming the Fear That Haunts Your Success* by P. R. Clance (1985).

2   I have achieved my other two dreams of being a writer (poetry, plays, many chemistry publications, and many psychotherapy books), and being a psychotherapist.

3   The basic Narrative Therapy premise is that "The person is not the problem, the problem is the problem." That is, their behavior is controlled by an internal entity that does not have their best interests in mind. So, the "cure" is to remove that entity so that it can no longer control their behavior. I used the word "exorcism" for the process of removing Peter's "a."

4   In the Gestalt Therapy (GT) training group I was in, and in other GT groups, it was not unusual for the leader to direct whoever was on the "hot seat" to go around the group, look each person in the eye, and make various statements. In such a group I would have asked Peter to say, "I used have performance anxiety. It is no longer here," to each person.

19 Case Study 12

Gloria and the Oboe and Being Adequate

> the notes flow outward
> so sonorously singing
> sliding to silence

Gloria plays the oboe and was the first oboist at an upcoming concert. She came to me because she said she would like to rid herself of almost paralyzing performance anxiety (PA). She has gotten good critiques from other musicians as to her playing. Her goal was being able to "play for fun." Gloria also told me that she had "angst about making mistakes forever." Also, a long time ago someone told her that she would always be just "adequate." So, my challenges were how to get her to be comfortable playing at the upcoming concert (three days away!), how to get rid of that old witch message of almost ever-present negative self-talk, and how to bring "fun" permanently back into her life. [She did tell me that there were times when playing oboe was fun, and not only in practicing, but also in occasional concerts. This told me that somehow and somewhere within her was the ability and capacity to be free of the old negativities.] Gloria also told me that she was a good percussionist, and this played a large part in what follows.

After a bunch of chatting, some of which was designed to "negate" the negative witch message, we then segued into a hypnosis session to establish rapport and provide information. The following has been reconstructed.

Well, Gloria, let's just start with your paying attention to your breathing. Just each breath, in and out, slowly, easily, naturally. One breath at a time, and one heartbeat. Continuing to breathe comfortably, you can just drift off within your mind to that special room in your home with your music and your oboe and your drums. Enjoy the familiarity of that room and all of the sounds that are somehow within it. That's a place where you can play to your heart's content, having your own kind of fun, knowing that you are really good and competent, and that you have had lots of good feedback from other musicians. That's right, is it not? They know a good professional musician from an amateur, do they not? Yes, and yes to that. And, you do know, do you not, the glory and wonder of making music with other professionals, all playing easily and comfortably together. The sounds from each of them and you just blend together, bringing the composer's magic with notes into a symphony of sound. Wow. And, you are happily part of that, all playing together under the conductor's guidance and baton. Little miracles like that happen, do they not?

And, now, something interesting is happening within you. There are the vibrations from my voice moving into you with words and ideas and sound sounds of calm and peace and confidence. At the same time, there in the background, and perhaps growing a bit softly louder, are some sounds of drumming. They are coming from your drums and afar, and carry with their vibrations, perhaps vibrations that are moving easily throughout your body and mind now, cleansing and cleaning out all of those old disturbing messages and thoughts and feelings. You may feel these vibrations loosening up that old stuff, and removing it permanently from your body and mind with each exhale, with each breath. So, that from now on you will be able to play your music with others, in concert with them, sharing with them, the joy of music, just vibrating forth into the concert hall. Wow. It is almost as if you were freed, really freed, completely and wholly freed. May I say "soundly" freed? Yes, and yes.

Continuing to breathe softly and easily and calmly. And, you know, Gloria, that you will be able to recall everything that has happened this afternoon whenever you need it, that's right, is it not? Just touch your ear now, and let that be a signal to remember these ideas and feelings and changes. So, any time in the future when you need to recall this, just briefly touch your ear, take a deep breath or two, and just have fun making music!

I want to thank you now for your trust and confidence and attention. And, whenever you are ready, just open your eyes, maybe blink a bit and stretch, and come back to this room here and now. Thank you.

Commentary

Gloria left looking quite relaxed and calm. She also appeared to be energized! Even though I have a "tin ear" and do not know much about music, it is always possible to work within the client's own special world. Let them take the lead.

20 Case Study 13

Nonagenarian Charlie with Anxiety about Eye Problem

> beneath the beech tree
> old man's beard sifting the sun
> insects flitter

I visited with an old friend of mine, Charlie, soon after his 91st birthday. [As is frequently the case with old friends, this was a *pro bono* visit. I offered to help him and he accepted.] He has had a bunch of eye problems, having lost sight in one eye about 50 years ago. Charlie is bright and active, very sociable, and a wonderful story teller. The remaining eye had a corneal transplant that was not healing well. So, Charlie was rather concerned and fearful and anxious about losing his eyesight. He was housebound and felt depressed. Guided imagery appeared to be the best way to help him at this time. Also, "normalizing" his feelings and state at this time was also appropriate so that he would be comfortable with the knowledge of his reaction being what anyone would feel. His GI choices are obvious in the following.

So, Charlie, we can just start with being comfortable in your easy chair, and just paying attention to your breathing. That's right, just breathing easily and comfortably in and out. With each inhale chest and belly softly rising, and with each exhale all of those muscles simply relaxing. Occasionally, a stray thought may wander through. Just thank it for being there, and go back to paying attention to your breathing.

Within your mind now you can just drift off and spend some time in your garden. You have always been a good gardener with oodles of flowers, and a green green lawn. A wonderful peaceful place to sit under a tree and read, look up at the sky and clouds, listen to birds, and notice the way that that gentle wind rustles through. That's right, continuing to breathe easily and normally there.

And now, something interesting happens. Your healer, Laura, slowly approaches. She is optimistic, encouraging, and upbeat. There has always been something special about her and being in her presence. She is close enough now to sit beside you and hold one of your hands. Before we started this I asked you if it would be okay for me to hold your hand. You said, "Yes."

So, I am reaching out now to hold your *other* hand. And now, somehow both through me and through Laura you are receiving healing energy and knowledge and ability. She knows just exactly where in your eye to send this healing and correcting energy. And right now, almost cell by cell, this is happening. To just bring your eye function back to normal, easily and simply. For you know that your body knows just how to do this. And, Laura is enhancing and empowering that ability so that sooner than you—or your doctor—would believe, you will be able for that eye to function normally and comfortably. Just one breath at a time. Perhaps one cell at a time. And organizing and reorganizing and strengthening your body's own healing systems. Yes, and yes, and yes. From us and through us, amazingly, simply and comfortably. And, gently, easily, naturally, Laura withdraws her hand as I do mine, yet you will retain that sense of our hands holding yours, will you not?

You know Charlie, that your body will retain what you have experienced this afternoon so that the healing work will continue easily and naturally, and soon your eye will be functioning normally. Good. Your doctor is very skilled and the healing has just taken a bit longer than you both may have expected. That is certainly within the normal range for this kind of procedure.

I want to thank you now for your trust and your confidence and your friendship. And, when you are ready, just take a deep breath or two, stretch a bit, and come back to this room here and now. Thank you.

[Sooner than he expected Charlie's eye was functioning properly again. He was quite relaxed at the end of the session. I heard from his daughter soon afterwards that he was back to his normal activities, and was driving again.]

21 Chatting Revisited

> Tell me and I'll forget. Show me and I may not remember.
> Involve me and I'll understand.
>
> (Native American Proverb)

21.1 Introduction

There appear to be over one zillion different ways to do therapy, and many of them are described by acronyms of several letters. I believe that the only one I seriously considered learning enough about to become sufficiently skilled in to use was NLP or Neurolinguistic Programming. I also became reasonably proficient in Ericksonian hypnosis and psychotherapy, Gestalt Therapy, Solution-Focused Therapy, Provocative Therapy, Logotherapy, Narrative Therapy, and Single-Session Therapy (SST) (to name a few) to use bits and pieces of them when working with clients. Out of curiosity, I also spent some time looking at and reading about some of the three- and four-letter therapies, although none of them convinced me to change how I work with clients. (Of course—being fairly ancient—I read Freud and others of his time. And, I must admit to having been in "analysis" for a number of years when I lived in Chicago. I will also admit that I have little "formal" training in any of the ways that I do therapy, having become skilled in many areas by reading and studying and practice and evaluating my practice.)

In 1978 I earned a master's degree in mental health counseling at Wright State University, and have been in private practice since that time (42 years). I have used many ways of doing psychotherapy and somehow I have evolved into chatting as my primary method.

At the present time there appears to be two ways of doing therapy: face-to-face (f2f) talk therapy, and non-present approaches including workbooks, online, and telephone. In my studies I have found that master therapists like Milton Erickson and Ernest Rossi emphasize face-to-face therapy since that allows them to read body language and *directly hear* all of the nuances in a client's speech. In observing a video or movie of Erickson or Rossi working with a volunteer or a client it is evident how closely they observe the client, are aware of movement and tone, and utilize their observations in their responses and interactions with the client. I have watched Rossi working with a volunteer whose eyes are closed and simply saying things like, "Yes, some more of that," "Stay with that," and "Just notice what is happening and where that moves." Rossi assumes the client knows and understands what "that" is. Obviously "that" is what the client is focused on at this moment. Wow! So, I am sold on f2f.

Clients come to us because they are stuck. That is, they have not been able to resolve the difficulties in their lives by themselves or by other helpers and therapists they have consulted. In some instances we become the helper of last resort. My published clinical case ("Mary and Anxiety and Insomnia and Shit and Einstein and …"—see Chapter 4) is relevant since Mary had been to many therapists and other helpers and finally(!) thought that hypnosis might help. Someone who knew of my work referred Mary to me. I generally work in the single-session mode, yet it took three sessions until Mary was satisfied that she had found what she wanted. In this section I am not writing about her, but something about being a therapist and how we work that has been of interest to me for a long time. When she came to see me she had been alive for over one half of one million hours. Lots and lots of living and memories and experiences. We were together for about four and one-half hours.

So, in the limited time we are f2f with a client how can we obtain any understanding of who they are and what they think and feel? How is it possible to establish a sufficiently trusting relationship so they openly share with us how they got to this point in their life where they are so stuck and blocked and even miserable? Somehow, in the way we greet them, ask questions, and listen, trust develops. In the literature this is called the " therapeutic alliance." And, the literature generally confirms that the therapeutic alliance is perhaps the most significant change agent in being a successful therapist.[1] (Of course, success is always the judgment of the client!) So, somehow in that 50 or 60 or 90 minutes contact is made, and the client is guided[2] to discover what it is they can do to get themselves out of their stuck place. Consider again that in the week before your client has come to see you (for those limited minutes) that they have been awake for about 112 hours. We then meet them in an isolated room for a tiny fraction of that week.

So, why have I emphasized above how limited is the time we have with a client with respect to their lives? My opening gambits are:

- Hi. You know that I work primarily as a single-session therapist. That is, I hope that in this session today whatever you have come to see me about will be resolved to your satisfaction. The choice is yours as to whether to come back for another session. Okay?
- Before we start, there is an interesting question that you can perhaps just let rattle around in your brain during the session. And that is, "What are you willing to change today?"

- So, what can I help you with today? That is, what has been bothering or troubling you or that you are so concerned about that you would like help with it? [Then I listen, take some notes, and make minor comments indicating that I have been listening! Like, "Okay," "Good," "Yes," "Interesting," and "Hmm."]

And, after this what I call "chatting" starts.

The basic idea is that two strangers have just met and they need to get to know each other. One way is to chat. You talk about common interests. Of course, this involves more self-disclosure than we have been taught to do, and which some therapists are uncomfortable doing. Yet, a connection is made. People always feel more at ease when they are with people like them, essentially those of the same background (ethnically, religiously, racially, professionally, etc.). So, there is some sharing of this. I have no preconceived expectation or agenda about where this chatting will go. At this point I may suggest an experiment of some kind or ask them to think about: (1) imagining that a miracle happened tonight, and that the miracle was that what they had come to consult me about would be completely and realistically resolved by tomorrow morning (the Miracle Question); (2) do you feel sometimes that you are being controlled by some sort of, perhaps, evil spirit inside you that takes over and sort of forces you to do things that are not helpful? (Narrative Therapy); (3) from what you have told me it seems that there are some unresolved issues between you and a significant person in your life, or that your mind is divided between making one of two choices, or that you feel trapped between two different feelings or ways of being (Gestalt Therapy Two-Chair Approach); and (4) do you feel that what is troubling you now, mental or physical, can be resolved or healed by some helping entity? (Guided Imagery). Generally, I *segue* via the chatting into one of these four approaches. Although I am experienced enough to guide the client via many other ways, these four approaches are the ones that I use most frequently.

Please note that all four of these approaches involve some level of hypnosis and trance states. That is, for example, when a client does the Gestalt Therapy two-chair procedure they become the two entities involved, and their language and demeanor change as they change chairs. In my experience, they get so involved in this role playing and so focused on what they are saying (effectively to themselves!) that they are in trance states. They frequently cannot recall what each part of them has said to the other, yet at the end they do recall and absorb the final rapprochement and agreements reached. There is relief and exhaustion, too. Also, (2) and (4) above incorporate hypnosis during the procedure.

When I use guided imagery I always ask if it turns out to be appropriate would it be okay if I hold one of their hands during that session. (I have yet to have this request refused, but I do not always do this—note the word "appropriate." The hand-holding has to be gentle and passive on my part.)

This occurs while the healing entity[3] is in contact with them (within their mind) or after the healing entity leaves. So, I will say, "I am reaching out to hold your hand now." And then I will say, "Somehow, somehow *from me and through me* you are also receiving whatever healing and help you need at this time." This contact can be quite significant as touch is so important, especially considering that when someone is in need contact with a healing person like a parent or nurse or spouse reaches parts of the mind/body that words do not. And, in another way, there is a built-in need for contact, a kind of regression to an almost primitive state that recalls childhood fears and hurts and pains. In the sentence in quotation marks above a critical word is "somehow" as it is sufficiently vague so that the client fills in whatever method of contact really reaches them. [In hypnosis and psychotherapy the words "yet" and "somehow" are a bit magical.]

Many NLP procedures incorporate anchors for particular mental and physical states, and for remembering. I find it useful in chatting to use anchors in two ways. The first way is to give themselves a signal (an anchor) to remind them of whatever occurred in the session that they need to remember or some action they need to take in certain circumstances. That is, something in their daily life would trigger the need to respond in a new and more helpful way. This anchor is a natural common movement like touching one's ear or nose or chin or perhaps bringing together some fingers. I then have them think about a time in the future where they would need to remind themselves of behaving or reacting differently, and then carrying out that movement. This is repeated two more times to reinforce the response and help to make it automatic. The second anchor is more "concrete" in the sense that I ask the client to pick a small smooth stone from my jar of stones. They keep the stone and touch it as they need to remind themselves of what they learned in the session that they would like to have occur in appropriate situations in the future.

The session ends with a continuation of the chatting with which it began, and a query about anything else they wish to discuss or bring up at this time. If appropriate, we shake hands or hug at the end of the session.

There may be many other therapists who "chat" with their clients, but who do not describe that they are working in that manner. I do know, for example, that when I have analyzed the clinical demonstrations I have observed at conferences that I have found that, no matter what the orientation of the demonstrator, it is generally possible to describe what they have done and are doing as either a variant of reframing or behavior modification. This all depends on your background and predilections. In this regard, I have been puzzled in the past in observing what Steve Gilligan does in his presentations and demonstrations, and in his writings. He is hugely respected for his skills. Yet, I have left one of these sessions or one of his books feeling that there is no way that I can figure out what he has done in a manner that I could incorporate it into my style. So, in writing and thinking about chatting in this chapter, I have come to the conclusion that Gilligan has his own style of chatting and being totally present with a client. The rapport (or therapeutic alliance if you will) is palpable in his easy style of just being with a client.

We also know from the literature on Erickson that he had an uncanny ability to be totally aware and present with a client—they knew that he was intensely focused on them and in a concerned and compassionate and sincere manner. In my hubris, perhaps, I could also describe Erickson as a chat-er!

Addendum May 6, 2019

Two days ago I met for the first time with a client I will call Elizabeth. She found me listed on the Internet as being a therapist in this area and was intrigued with what was written there. Elizabeth is in her early 70s, is retired, and has worked in the mental health field for many years. She is divorced, overweight, and is searching for meaning in her life. She came to the session with two pages of prepared comments about what was going on in her life at this time, and what she hoped I could help her with. After listening to her opening statement and making appropriate notes and comments to indicate that I was listening and following what she said, we chatted for a bit with my responding to her questions about myself and what I did, and sharing with her some similarities in our work and backgrounds.

[I did start off the session with comments about how I worked in terms of single-session therapy, and that she had the option of requesting additional sessions, asking her if it would be okay to hold a hand if that was appropriate (she said Yes), and to just keep in the back of her mind somewhere Mary Goulding's opening question of "What are you willing to change today?"] I also thought that both the Miracle Question and my approach called Guided Metaphor, which I use to help clients who are having a global need for changing their lives and finding meaning in them, would be appropriate. It was also understood that if it was useful to use hypnosis, that I would do so. Before launching into the Miracle Question I spent about five minutes going over the basics of weight control since this was something she was concerned about. She understood the need to decrease caloric intake as well as increase exercise. I also urged her to get her medical doctor to prescribe a course of physical therapy for the physical difficulties she had been having.]

So, I suggested that she close her eyes and led her through the Miracle Question. Elizabeth initially responded with some post-miracle comments, but then did not continue. Since she appeared to be in a light trance and was relaxed, I decided to segue into the guided imagery format with initial comments about drifting off in her mind to a safe and secure and special place that was hers. Elizabeth is a member of a special religious group, and I then suggested that she could sense the presence of one of the prophets of that group coming near her, and then gently touching her. (I did not hold her hand during this session.) Via that touch He was transferring to her whatever internal strength and knowledge and change she needed realistically at this time of her life. I spent several minutes with much detail on the things that were being transferred to her so that she would find meaning in her life and calmness and peace. Earlier she had told me about a man holding open a door for her and giving her a *genuinely* rich smile when she said "Thank you." So, I had her healer also smile. I ended in my usual way of reminding her she could re-experience what she had learned this afternoon and the time with the healer whenever she needed this. There was an "aura" of peace about Elizabeth at the end of the session. At that time I showed her my jar of polished stones and told her she should take one as a gift and reminder of what had occurred this afternoon. She chose one and was touched by the "gift."

Commentary

I include the description of this session here as another reminder of how effective I feel that "chatting" can be with clients. Chatting is almost the essence of establishing the therapeutic alliance, is it not? Isn't this what you do with chance encounters on airplanes or other occasions? Chatting for me means really being there with a client in an interpersonal encounter where we both know that the our mutual goal is to explore and find ways that whatever has been troubling him or her will realistically and satisfactorily be resolved. I believe that this way of interacting (and it is an interaction) is conducive to rapid change.

Finally, may I opine here that I think that Elizabeth will call for another session some time. [I did smile and shake her hand when she left.]

Notes

1 In most of the training workshops I have conducted (and some of my books) there is a section on rapport building. These are the "tricks" of the trade that lead to a client's being comfortable and trusting. I cannot overestimate the importance of *subtly* establishing rapport.

2 I prefer nowadays to consider myself as being a "guide" to the client's own inner resources. This is the belief of many therapists (and mine) that the client already knows and has the ability of what to do to bring about desired realistic change(s) in his/her life.

3 I am deliberately vague about the nature of the "healing entity" for I want my client to choose who and what that is. This becomes clear to me sometimes, and sometimes it does not. Yet, it is *their* healing entity that is important.

22 Case Study 14

Joe and the NLP Fast Allergy Cure

> glistening grass
> sheening for the morning's sun
> a spider's web, too

A long time ago, I learned about the NLP (Neurolinguistic Programming) fast allergy cure. At that time I carried out a short research project with about eight people I knew who had allergies. I do not recall how many I was able to help then, but I was surprised (although I shouldn't have been!) that subject A was allergic to goldenrod and not cat dander or tree pollens and that subject B was allergic to tree pollens but not cat dander or goldenrod. So, allergies are highly specific. In researching allergies I came across an early study in Vienna of a doctor finding that his patient (who was allergic to roses) started sneezing when she came into his office where he had some artificial roses! This indicated that there was a psychological aspect to allergies. Well, if that were the case, then allergies might be cured by a psychological intervention (such as the NLP one).

For this case study I start with a reconstructed transcript of a session with my friend Joe (this was *pro bono*) who had had allergies since he was three or four. They were mostly fall pollens and dust, and occasionally spring pollens. After the description of that session (which was successful and took about 20 minutes), I will list the steps of the NLP fast allergy cure with appropriate commentary.

22.1 NLP Fast Allergy Cure with Joe

Joe, I would like to sit close enough to you to touch some knuckles on your hand. Would that be okay? [Yes.] While I touch this knuckle, just go inside your mind and think about a recent time when you were in the presence of one of these allergens and had a small reaction. [I do not want a strong reaction, since I want to calibrate that just thinking about being in the presence of the allergen produces the response so I can anchor it, and check later if thinking about the allergen still produces a reaction.] Thank you. That is just enough [and I stop touching that knuckle]. I explained earlier that an allergic reaction is just a learned mistake of the immune system. Somewhere and some time in your past your immune system made the mistake of not ignoring an allergen, or a group of allergens, so that you ended up being sensitive to them. I also told you how it is possible—as I just demonstrated—that thinking about being in the presence of the allergen can produce a reaction. So, there is a psychological aspect to allergic reactions, which is why the procedure we are going to go through today can eliminate that reaction. Okay? [Nods yes.]

Now [touching a different knuckle], it would be helpful at this time for you to think about some recent time or times when you were really feeling good about yourself, competent and healthy. Let me know when you have found such a time or times. [Nods yes, and I add a little pressure to the knuckle to anchor that so that he will have a sense of being in charge and okay during the following.]

There is one more thing we need to find out about at this time and that is what we call a counter example. That is, all of the allergens you are sensitive to are small, dust-like particles. Is there something like that to which you are not sensitive? [Thinks, says yes.] What is it? [Well flour, like used in baking, is like that and I have no problem around flour.] Thank you.

The room we are in now is a relatively small one. I'd like you to imagine now and see in front of you a transparent, perhaps glass or plexiglass partition, that goes from ceiling to floor and wall to wall. Okay? [Thinks for a moment, and nods Yes.] Just imagine now that you can see out there on the other side of that transparent barrier a younger you, perhaps two years old, and before the time that your immune system made those mistakes. He is playing there with some flour and water. He is happily doing that. And, you notice that he is out of doors where there are trees and grass and some dust blowing about. They do not bother him at all. His immune system is working perfectly well. [Touching another knuckle.]

And, now, something interesting happens. He turns and looks at you, and you look at him. The transparent barrier slowly and simply dissolves and disappears. That younger you gets up, comes closer to you, and you reach out and hold hands with him. You are holding both hands. And, at this time, somehow, somehow, there is a transfer of knowledge and ability and information from that younger you's immune system to yours. You might even feel a kind of tingling sensation at this time with that contact, from his hands. So that, somehow, he is making a gift to you of your old immune system's ability to ignore and counteract and make ineffective any allergic reaction to the things that had mistakenly troubled you all these years. Your immune system is now fully functioning, is it not? Good.

Within your mind now thank that younger you for his gift, and just feel and imagine hugging that younger you. His immune system is diffusing within your body and merging with yours and freeing you from those past mistakes. Slowly, easily, naturally, completely and comfortably. And, again, thank that younger you for this gift.

[Holding the resource anchor and lightly touching the allergy reaction anchor, I observed Joe. There were no allergic reactions at this time. He continued to breath easily and comfortably.] I am going to remove my hand now, and want you to know that your immune system has now learned how to ignore those allergens, and that you will be okay from this time on. With your younger you's gift in mind, just think now about sometime soon when you would be in the presence of those things that used to trouble you. [He does so, and there is no reaction.] Thank you.

Joe, you will remember what has happened here this afternoon. Sometimes, permanent changes like this really happen this fast. Keep in touch. [On later contact, Joe reported that he continued to be free of these allergic reactions.]

Here is a list of the steps involved:

1   Start with explaining that allergies are a mistake of the immune system and that there is a psychological component to allergies. This establishes the physiological and psychological bases for the NLP approach. Find out when and where the allergy started, i.e., what age and the location if that is relevant. What is the client allergic to (may be one thing, one class of things, or a number of them)?

2   Calibrate the allergic response by setting an anchor and observing the client's reactions when s/he thinks about being in an environment where the allergen(s) is/are present. Remove the anchor touch once the reaction is observed, and remember how you set it so you can test at the end of the session.

3   Anchor a resource state, i.e., recent times when they have felt okay about themselves and in charge. Maintaining this resource and feeling okay about yourself state throughout the process enhances the changes that occur. It is a protective action.

4   Suggest counter examples to the allergen, that is, substances that are similar (small particles, e.g.) but to which the client shows no allergic reactions. In the case written about above, baking flour is made up of small particles.

5   Have the client imagine that the room they are in has a transparent partition in it (glass or plexiglass) separating the room into two parts.

6   Then, have the client imagine seeing their younger self (a year or two younger than the age the allergy started) on the other side of the partition. Their younger self is in the presence of the allergen(s), but does not react to them. The younger self's immune system has not been "fooled" by the allergen(s), and they do not bother him/her at all.

7   The younger and current self see each other, the barrier slowly disappears, the younger self draws closer and they touch holding hands. There is now a *transfer* of the younger self's intact and functioning immune system to the current self via the contact. That is, *somehow* (magic word!) the current immune system is learning and storing how not to be fooled by the allergen(s), so they will no longer have any effect.

8   Then the older self thanks the younger self for this gift, hugs him/her, and somehow the younger self diffuses into the older self's body and mind and immune system, so that its intact and effective immune system has now become a fully integrated part of the older person. Again, the older self thanks the younger one for this gift.

9   The resource anchor, which has been held all of this time, is gently removed, and the client is returned to the here and now.

10   The final part of this process is to test the changes by touching the anchor set at the beginning for the client reacting to the allergen(s). Assuming the process has worked, the client will show no allergic symptoms. Another test that can be performed at this time is to ask the client to imagine being in the presence of the allergen(s) at some time in the future, and note their response.

Commentary

I have used this with quite a few clients with remarkable success. The entire procedure generally takes 20–30 minutes.

23 Case Study 15

Joan and the NLP VK Dissociation Fast Phobia Cure

in the eastern sky
above twilight cloud wisps
half moon hanging

When I was studying NLP a long time ago (and also teaching about it) one of the interventions I came across was the VK dissociation fast phobia cure (see Andreas, 2014b). One of the first people I helped using this approach was a friend of ours named Joan who had a fear of flying. The NLP premise is that phobias are triggered by a person seeing something in their environment (V for visual) and then having a physical (K for kinesthetic) response. This response is usually manifested as one of panic with all of its physiological components. So, the procedure is to separate or unlink or dissociate the kinesthetic response from the visual one. The entire procedure usually takes about 20 minutes. The NLP premise is that phobias begin with a single (scary) incident some time back when they were much younger. Then, if the person learned how to be phobic that quickly, they can also learn to *not* respond to that stimulus in a single session. Before giving a reconstructed transcript of the process I will present the step-by-step treatment procedure.[1]

1 First establish a strong and reliable resource for the person and anchor it (by touching a place on her knee or shoulder). That is, she needs to be in a stable and resourceful state.
2 Get a small indication of the phobic response by having her think about a situation where she would be in the presence of the phobic stimulus. Anchor this response, and be sure that you ask for only a *brief and small* interaction.
3 Have her visualize being in a large but empty movie theater with the screen somewhere out in front of her.
4 While holding the resource anchor, have her go back to just *before* the original traumatic incident that started this phobic response, and see herself up on the screen in black and white as a still slide or photograph. [A phobic response almost always has a memorable first time.]

5   She then floats out of the picture to see herself in the audience. [This makes a contact between the person on the screen and the one in the audience.]
6   She then floats out of herself to see herself in the audience, perhaps from somewhere behind her (could be the projection booth).
7   At this point, she imagines being in the projection booth (or behind somewhere) watching herself in the audience watching the screen. [This creates a *double dissociation*. That is, the person is not watching the screen directly, but is watching themselves watching the screen.]
8   While dissociated in this way, she can watch herself watching the movie of the traumatic incident.
9   She watches the movie from up in the safety of the projection booth until it moves forward until the end of the incident. Then she can watch the movie from the beginning again from her protected position.
10   When the movie is finished (and still holding the resource anchor), she can float down from the projection booth to her seat in the audience.
11   Then, float from the audience onto the screen at the end of the movie and run it backwards associated with her image on the screen *very fast backwards*. [Note: this entire process can be run several tries as needed until her emotions have flattened out—monitor her breathing and affect.]
12   Finally, test by firing the phobia anchor you set at the beginning of this process. [Assuming that she got into all of the phases of this process, there will be no indications of a phobic state. The key is to dissociate emotional kinesthetic responses from visual ones.]

23.1 Joan and Fear of Flying

Joan was one of the first people I ever worked with using the VK dissociation method for phobias, and this was about 35 years ago in New Zealand. This worked in one session with her, and I know this since she and her husband flew many places afterwards, including the U.S. where we met up with them twice when he was here as a visiting professor. Here is a reconstruction for the process as I recall using it at that time (it is slightly different than the one outlined above).

RUBIN (R):   First I need just a little bit of information about your fear of flying. I believe you said earlier that you were okay with flying for a while, but then this fear developed.
JOAN (J):   That's right.
R: When did this start, and how old were you then?
J: It was in 1975 and I was 35 years old then.
R: Was there some particular incident that triggered this?

J: We were flying home and hit a bunch of turbulence, and I just had this panic that the plane would crash.

R: You did land safely then, didn't you?

J: Yes.

R: Good. To go through this process comfortably and safely it would be useful now if you were to close your eyes and just think about some time recently when you were feeling good about yourself, when you were in charge and just feeling okay. [She closes her eyes.] I am just going to reach over now and touch your shoulder if that is okay. [Nods yes, and I set an anchor for this resource state.]

R: [While holding this anchor I say ...] At this time I want to just check on that phobia. So, just think briefly and a little bit about being in an airplane. Thank you. That is enough. [I set another anchor for the phobic state and then remove it as she calms down. This anchor, of course, is used later to check on the phobia.]

R: Now, remaining calm and comfortable, just imagine that you are in an empty movie theater sitting somewhere near the middle or back. Let me know when you are there. [Nods.] Up on the screen in front of you, you can now see a still slide or photograph of yourself some time before that incident started, and you were comfortably in your seat in the airplane. You may be looking out of the window or reading, and you can even see what you were wearing at that time, can you not? [Nods yes.] Thank you. Now, just kind of float out of yourself so you can see yourself sitting there and looking at that photo. Good. Continue floating safely until you are in the projection booth behind the glass there. And, you can now look down and see yourself sitting in the theater as she looks at the screen. From the projection booth looking past yourself in your seat a movie starts showing that time when all of this started. Look at that movie until it ends, and then run it quickly back to before the event started. Thank you. Once again, let that movie run forward, perhaps a bit more swiftly this time, until it ends. Then it runs rapidly backwards to well before this all started. To be sure about all of this, watch again from up in the projection booth, past yourself down in the theater, the movie running to its end, and then returning to before it begins. Now, the screen blacks out as you float back into yourself sitting in the theater. [Of course, holding the resource anchor all of this time, and making a gentle increase in pressure if you notice any emotional response.]

R: Well, Joan, you can just return to here and now, perhaps just stretching a bit and blinking your eyes. Thank you. [She opens her eyes and looks at me. At this point I trigger the anchor for the phobic response and observe. Nothing happens.] What was that like for you?

J: It was interesting watching myself watch that movie. In the end it all just seemed to disappear somehow.

R: Interesting. [Continuing to lightly hold the resource anchor ...] Joan, just think now about getting on plane and flying somewhere. Okay? [She does.] You're smiling!

J: Yes. It feels okay. I know that the planes are safe and that the pilots are well-trained. The planes are really designed to shake, aren't they?

R: Yes. [We both laugh a little.] The interesting thing, Joan, about phobias is that people learn quickly usually from a single incident to be scared of something. So, if they are able to learn quickly how to be scared, then they can learn just as quickly—as you did now—to get over that. The mind is really remarkable.

J: Thank you.

Note

1   The VK dissociation basic phobia treatment procedure is described on the web as well as in many books.

24 Healing Factors

calm morning sun
sharp shadows slant towards me
one bright ray

24.1 Introduction

Starting with a number of useful opening statements by several therapists that I use as appropriate:

- "What are you willing to change today?" (Mary Goulding)
- "When are you able to control the problem rather than it controlling you?" (Michael White)
- "Please do not tell me anything you do not wish to tell me." (Milton H. Erickson)
- "Whenever I have an hypothesis about what is going on in my client, I lie down until it goes away." (Bill O'Hanlon)
- "When patients come into my office, I greet them with a blank mind and I look them over to see who and what and why they are without taking anything for granted." (Milton H. Erickson)

Next are two useful bits of information from the Brief Family Therapy Center of Milwaukee:

A. Three Types of Clients

- Workers—are ready and willing to change.
- Complainants—there to complain, but can be helped to become a worker.
- Visitors—mandated to be there by someone in the family or the legal system. Rarely able to get them to work. Mainly, just be friendly with them. [Occasionally, visitors can be helped.]

[Note: would you rather spend time with a complainer or someone who is describing what works and has worked for them?]

B. Fundamental Three Rules for Doing Therapy

- If it is not broken, don't fix it.
- If it worked once, do it again.
- If it doesn't work, don't do it again. Do something different.

There are five factors in the literature that appear to support spontaneous remissions and healing. They are:

- Being married.
- Having a support network.
- Having a strong religious or spiritual faith.
- Having a goal and meaning in life.
- Being a "fighter"—being active vs. being passive.

Alternative or complementary therapies are quite popular. There appear to be at least a zillion of them that people have tried and used. There is a continuing and huge market for vitamins and supplements and special diets. Almost every study I have read about taking these wonderful pills and powders have found them to be mostly worthless and just enriching your eliminations. Here are some comments about alternative and complementary therapies (Anonymous, 1992).[1] In this 1992 book there is a long list of expert contributing editors and contributors. We summarize their key findings in the following six bullets:

- All of the alternative/complementary therapies discussed in this book have worked for someone.
- The essence of effectiveness is the *placebo effect*, that is, do they believe in it?
- There is some evidence that acupuncture, Chinese medicine, and hypnosis work.
- Ask what users feel, sense, and believe will work for them.
- Religion is very important to some people.
- There are many "fads" like coffee enemas that have been used over time.

The contributors to this volume searched for research studies on all of the topics discussed and evaluated in the book. Only the three mentioned in the third bullet appeared to have some validity.

Finally, under healing factors it is important to know that you do have under your control the following seven items: environment, treatments, personnel, relationships, time, activities, and how you respond. That is, there are many decisions relating to your physical and mental health that are within your power to make.

24.2 Acting As-If as a Healing Factor

A number of years ago I had a new client whose opening comment was something like, "Two weeks ago I decided to be happy, and since then I have been happy. That is not what I have come to see you about." So, we worked on something else. The amazing part of this for me was that in the two sessions I saw her that what she ended up telling me about her life (before the decision to be happy) had enough ups and downs and crazy things in it to provide plots for at least a dozen soap operas. The issues that she did bring up were resolved to her satisfaction in those two sessions.

Spending time with her opened up new vistas for me. (Just think of how much we have learned from our clients, and how they have inspired us to explore new avenues!) Mary Goulding's opening query of "What are you willing to change today?" almost implies "What are you willing to act As-If it was different in your life?" When you think about this, is it not the essence of what we do as therapists? That is, providing the opportunity for and facilitating their discovering different and more appropriate ways to live their lives. Perhaps this can be implemented by simply telling the story about the "happy" client and asking, "What are you willing to decide today that will resolve realistically and to your satisfaction what it is that you have come to see me about?" This question would be enhanced by adding, "Do not make that decision right now, just let it float around in the back of your mind during this session." This is what is usually called "seeding." Imagine seeding in this way at the beginning of a session rather than starting with collecting a lot of information via the standard history.

Acting As-If is a variant of reframing or using a crystal ball to look back from the future or using the Miracle Question. And, metaphors can be considered to be ways of imagining and experiencing other (As-If) ways of being and living. To continue these ideas we can consider all embedded suggestions (via hypnosis or other approaches) to actually be a form of psychological placebo effect. Recall that in medicine the placebo effect is believing that an inert substance actually has medicinal results, and that in psychotherapy suggestions actually have behavioral results. That is, in essence, the client in a psychotherapy session expects and believes that the words used by the therapist will change their lives in the ways that they desire.

With all of the preceding in mind in this section I present a number of approaches to changing behavior related to As-If that my friend and colleague Trevor Silvester describes in his book *Cognitive Therapy* (2010). We'll start with the Gestalt Therapy two-chair method where the client acts As-If he/she can talk with another person or another part of themselves. Silvester writes:

> The success of the Gestalt Chair technique depends on several factors. The first is that it is only as good as the involvement of the client. They have to

speak to the other person [or part of themselves] as if that other person was actually there, and when they are the other person they need to speak in the first person. ... I'll often encourage them to adopt the physiology of the other person: it really helps them to "get in character."

The second point is to remember what the exercise is there to achieve. ...

(p. 171)

[There are two questions to keep in mind.] "What is it the client needs to say to X, that by saying it will mean they can let go of the problem?" and "What is it the client needs to hear from X, that by hearing it will mean they can let go of the problem?"

(p. 172)

The therapist guides the client in these exchanges in terms of suggesting questions (to both parts) and telling the client when to switch chairs. In my experience a resolution is reached in 10–15 minutes via 8 to 10 exchanges. It is useful noting that clients appear to act As-If they were the person in the other chair, and often appear to be in a hypnotic state. Also, this is one of the most frequent approaches I use in a variety of circumstances.

With regard to As-If here are some more useful comments on pp. 220–221 (Silvester, 2010):

Adopting the physiology of a state tends to lead to the experience of the state. Welcome to the science of "fake it until you make it." ... Can I ask you to adopt the physiology of a depressed person for a moment? Feel how your state declines as you do so. Conversely, stand or sit like you're confident. Again, calibrate that feeling. We intuitively know what goes with what: the physiology has a correlate in the mind to a state or emotion. *Our physiology dictates our state and our state dictates what's on our mind.* [emphasis added]

Another insightful comment (p. 222) is, "most therapy happens in between sessions. By giving them things they can do for themselves it helps to reinforce their internal locus of control and create a sense of empowerment." (Related to this is Milton Erickson's simple approach of getting clients to do one thing in their life differently.) Lastly, in this paragraph, is an observation about Positive Psychology (p. 224),

Seligman's (2003) moment of genius was to realize what an untapped resource were people living happy, fulfilled lives. Positive Psychology became the study of positive emotions, positive traits and strengths, and positive institutions. Its research has shown that happiness, positivity and optimism increase health, longevity and quality of life, and people can take active steps to increase their default setting for optimism. A lot of it is managing the way you think of your future, because *we tend to get the future we expect.* [emphasis added]

Here are four exercises that Silvester obtained from Positive Psychology that are related to As-If:

- Gratitude: Find three opportunities in a day to thank somebody for something—beyond the run of everyday pleasantries.
- Savoring: we live in such a fast pace that we can go a surprisingly long time without appreciating the moment. Either set aside a period of minutes every day, or choose two or three times per day, and *savor* them.
- Kindness: Do an act of random kindness every day. Do it with no thought of personal gain, and do it at some cost or inconvenience to you if possible.
- Are You in Growth or Protection?: Ask yourself questions like, "Which decision keeps us in growth?" or "Are we in growth or protection?" or "Where is that decision coming from?"

Note

1 Much of this information has come from this source. Although this is an old report it is full of common sense and was a thorough study of the literature at that time.

25 Guided Imagery, Hypnosis, and Other Approaches for Palliative Care

the cry of a crow
floats higher than the mountain
a stream rushes down

25.1 Palliative Care, Comfort Care, and Hospice Care

The primary goal of *palliative care* is to help people with serious diseases feel better. That is, it focuses on relieving suffering and improving every day functioning. It is not on curing the disease, but rather prevents or treats symptoms and the side effects of the disease and its treatments. The goal of *comfort care* is more modest in the sense that it is to help everyone involved feel more comfortable, that is, not only the gravely ill, but also family members, medical personnel, and nursing home staff.

Hospice care was initially both the philosophy and practice of attending to the physical, emotional, medical, and spiritual needs of people approaching the end of life. In recent times, hospice care has included many aspects of palliative care. In the U.S., hospice care is a medical benefit available to anyone who has less than six months to live if their medical condition follows its natural course and two physicians certify that this is the case. This care can be at home or in a nursing home. There are both nonprofit and for profit hospice services. (See https//:hospicecarefoundation.org.) There are four levels of hospice care, and these are evaluated for need by hospice caregivers. The first level includes such things as: skilled nursing services, physical and occupational therapy, medical social services, home health aide services, medical supplies and durable medical equipment. In level 2, continuous home care is available during times of crisis or when a higher level of continuous care is needed. Inpatient care is provided (level 3) when symptoms cannot be treated at home. This may be at a free-standing hospice facility or in a nursing home. Respite care (level 4) is provided for caregivers for no more than five days with the patient in an incare facility. (Sadly, many patients and their families wait too long to obtain hospice services.)

The main differences between hospice care and palliative care are (note that both are provided wherever in most communities):

- Palliative care does not require a six month prognosis for life.
- In palliative care a patient can continue to receive treatments to cure their illness, while hospice care only provides symptom relief.
- The amount and duration of palliative care you receive depends on your medical insurance plan.

It is important to note that palliative care is provided in hospitals, outpatient clinics, nursing homes, or at home. Most important is that palliative care is a *multidisciplinary team effort* involving doctors, nurses, psychologists, psychiatrists, social workers, massage therapists, physical and occupational therapists, nutritionists, and chaplains. In essence, it deals with end-of-life care, and dealing with the distress of physical or psychosocial or spiritual pain. At the present time there are over 1700 hospitals in the U.S. with more than 50 beds that have a palliative care team (this is 72% of such U.S. hospitals, and they serve 87% of all hospitalized patients in the U.S.).[1]

25.2 Guided Imagery and Palliative Care

Guided imagery can be a powerful method for providing palliative care. In the following two scripts—one for palliative care, the other for healing—both can be used with individuals or groups. In your delivery *include many pauses* to allow the listener to fill in his/her own memories and details. There are many words and phrases that can be subtly emphasized to initiate memories or internal searches, and also mark out specific suggestions (a few are indicated in italics). It is assumed in the following that suggesting that the listener(s) begin the relaxation portion of the session by paying attention to their breathing is an effective and common way to start. For some patients it may be important to first describe what a guided imagery session is like in terms of starting with relaxation, and followed by just talking about ways that provide comfortable and useful ways of thinking about themselves and their situation.

A. Script for Guided Imagery for Palliative Care

So, let's just begin with your finding a way to be comfortable in that chair, knowing that you can move around at any time to be more comfortable. That's right. And, we can just start with paying attention to your breathing. Just notice each breath as it comes in and goes out, slowly, easily, naturally. And, with each inhale chest and belly are softly rising. Then, with each exhale, all of those muscles are just relaxing. You can even imagine that each inhale is a kind of energizing and healing breath, while each exhale is a kind of cleansing and clearing breath. Just one breath at a time. One heartbeat. From time to time a stray thought may wander through, just notice it, thank it for being there, and go back to this breath, and the next one. This is your time now. Feel free to change what I say to whatever you need now and that *will be helpful* to you at this time of your life. This breath and the next one.

And, within your mind now, you can just drift off to some special place that is uniquely yours, a healing and learning and safe and secure place. It may be real or imaginary, this special place. *Enjoy being there.* Just look around and sense around your own special place. I don't know where it is or what it is like, you do, do you not? This breath and the next one.

Something interesting now happens while you safely think about what is going on in your life at this time. Much is changing and has changed, has it not? Life is just different, and there may be too many new things going on. Yet, you are still you, are you not? And, this sense of who you are is deep inside you, helping you cope and adjust to all of the changes. In what came before you may have encountered a number of challenges that you managed to get through. Yes and yes. Sometimes with the help of others, and sometimes by yourself. This breath and the next one. So, you have learned much in your life and done many things. From time to time you may find yourself thinking about your life and what you have done, the sad times and the happy ones. And, here you are now, facing new challenges and learning how to cope and adapt with the help and guidance and support of this special group. Continuing to breathe comfortably and easily.

One thing you may have learned already is that you can give a person a gift by asking them to help you. We have all been taught to help others, have we not? Yet, giving them the opportunity to help us is really a gift. It is really really a gift to ask for help and assistance. Just think about that for a while. And, sharing openly with some people can be helpful, too. You know and I know that there are those you can share with, and those to just ignore in this way. A friend once told me that he would say when asked how he was, "I'm okay, there is just something wrong in my body." He was a pretty wise guy, wasn't he?

This breath and … There are so many ways to learn. Another friend told me that he never learned what love really was until he got sick. It is interesting that so much changes, so much does not, and that love and friendship endure to sustain us. Lots of things to think about now.

You know that your mind can remember what we have talked about today. So, if you need to recall these feelings and ideas, all you need to do is to find a quiet place, pay attention to your breathing, and you will remember and recall all of the helpful feelings and ideas. I want to thank you for your trust and attention. And when you are ready, just take a deep breath or two, blink your eyes, stretch a bit, and come back to this room here and now. Thank you.

Just one thing more. I have here a jar that has a bunch of small polished stones in it. Please pick one to take with you to remember this session.

Commentary

Guided imagery sessions are typically 15 minutes. The language used here can be used for one person or a group. However, if you are working with one person, it is useful to find out how they relax (or meditate), what their "safe haven" is, and also who or what will help them through their current difficult times. Also, the gift of one of the small polished stones is a *solid* reminder of the session.

A person who is in a palliative care program has a serious chronic or life-challenging illness. Since guided imagery was originally developed to work with people who had cancer, and with the belief that envisioning healing and/ or curing possibilities, the following script is designed towards those ends. It is designed for working with a group.

B. Guided Imagery Script for Healing

This guided imagery session is designed to enhance and use your own mental and physical resources to minimize the effects and progress of your illness. It has also been known to lead to cures or greatly reduce the extent of an illness. A good way to start on this healing journey is to get relaxed. So, please find a way to be comfortable in your chair knowing that you can shift positions to be more comfortable at any time. We can begin with your paying attention to your breathing. Just notice each breath as it goes in and goes out. Softly, easily, naturally. And, each inhale is a kind of energizing and enabling breath. Each exhale is a kind of cleansing and clearing breath. Just one breath at a time, one heartbeat. With each inhale chest and belly softly rising, and then with each exhale all of those muscles just relaxing. This breath, and the next one.

And, within your mind now, just drift off to some special place that is uniquely yours. It may be real or imaginary. This is a learning and healing place. Enjoy being there. Perhaps, you even look around that place reliving special memories and feelings. It's a place where you are protected and comfortable, a healing place. This breath and the next one.

And now, something interesting happens—you become aware that somewhere near you is a powerful healer or energy. I do not know exactly who or what this healer is or what the healing energy source is like, yet you do have a sense right now about this, do you not? This healing power comes closer to you and gently makes contact. It is both knowledgeable and powerful. Then, somehow, somehow, through this contact it is empowering your immune system and healing faculties to become more effective, more efficient, and more capable of improving your health slowly, easily, and in a natural way.

You can almost sense, can you not, that somehow each cell and tissue and organ and nerve in your body and your mind is becoming more knowledgeable and effective in healing you. Slowly and easily and naturally. One part of you at a time. This breath and the next one. This heartbeat. You may even sense somewhere within you, and maybe many places, that these changes are already occurring and have occurred. And, within your mind now, you thank this healing power or force or entity for this gift. This breath and the next one. Then, slowly, it moves away since it has more work to do, more people to help.

Continuing to breathe easily and normally. I want to thank you for your trust and your attention. And, whenever you are ready, just take a deep breath or two, blink your eyes, stretch a little bit, and come back to this room here and now. Thank You. [A stone is offered to the client at the end of the session.]

Commentary

Again, this is a kind of generic and general guided imagery for healing. If you are working with a group, you can ask them what kind of healer or force or power they would prefer—I generally give a group three choices: healing light, healing touch, or a healer. Then I use that in the session. In working with an individual it is important to find out *their* preferred safe haven and healing entity and something about each of these aspects. [Belleruth Naparstek sells many guided imagery CDs for different conditions and purposes: www. healthjourneys.com.]

25.3 Psychotherapy for Palliative Care

My volunteer work for over three decades has been with caregivers and people who have life-challenging diseases. The Charlie Brown support group described in Chapter 2 is effectively group therapy, although for people who could also be in a palliative care program. I was always careful to *not do* individual therapy in that group since it was the *group* therapy that helped them. The group had a lending library of recordings and books and pamphlets. My most recommended books were (I believe they would all be of some use to patients in palliative care):

- All of Bernie Siegel's books (see references), especially his first book (1986), *Love, Medicine & Miracles.*
- Stephen Schneider's *The Patient from Hell* (2005) whose subtitle accurately describes the book—"How I worked with my doctors to get the best of modern medicine and how you can too."

- Alison Shapiro's *Healing into Possibility*. (2009) The subtitle is "The transformational lessons of a stroke." She describes how she worked back to health from two strokes via intense dedication to her recovery.
- Rachel Naomi Remen's *Kitchen Table Wisdom* (1996). This is a remarkable collection of healing stories.
- Stephen Levine's *A Year To Live* (1997) in which he describes living his life *as if* he had only one year more to live.

Chapter 3 has material on using hypnosis for preparing patients for surgery, and this should be considered for palliative care patients. In the next section I reprise the part of Chapter 3 having to do with variations of Remen's healing circle approach as applied specifically to palliative care and other areas.

25.4 Variations of the Remen Healing Circle for Palliative Care Patients and Related Groups

This variation of Remen's healing circle can be applied to palliative care groups, assisted living facility groups, sentient residents of nursing homes, residents of ReHab units, and sentient residents of hospice facilities (see more details in section 3.2B). The groups would consist of a facilitator and four to eight people, with six being a good number. They all use a bowl of small polished variegated stones. A meeting would focus on one especially needy and designated person in the group or the entire group as follows.

A. Focused on One Member

This person would briefly describe to the group what is going in their life, and what is their special need for support. This may be depression, anxiety, stress, pain, or something else. To enhance sharing everyone in the group agrees that whatever is said in the group is strictly confidential and will not be told to anyone else. The volunteer picks a stone up from the bowl. This stone is passed around the group and each person in the group holds the stone up and briefly tells how they personally coped with the presented difficulty or condition. At the end of their relevant personal story they say, "I put courage/strength/love/God/Jesus/family/children/Nature into this stone for you," and then pass it on. The stone is then given to the central person to keep. The stone then becomes a kind of sacred power and enhancing amulet or talisman for the recipient. (Some people have a small ring cemented to the stone and wear it using a chain.)

A feature of this group activity is that each person who shares their personal story in the group also hears what others have done to help themselves through a difficult situation or emotional crisis. So, they are all connected and have learned different ways of coping.

B. Focused on the Entire Group

The session is focused on a particular topic like coping with anxiety, depression, pain, grief, stress, or something else. Each person in the group picks a stone from the bowl. Then, one by one, they hold the stone up and briefly share how they coped with that difficulty. That is, what personal activity or characteristic helped them through that time. At the end they say, "I put (the activity or characteristic) in this stone for everyone." When they have spoken (this may include the facilitator), the facilitator asks them to put their stone back in the bowl, mixes up all of the stones, and then asks each member to pick up a different stone from the bowl. Assuming the chairs in the room are close enough, each person holds their stone in their right hand and they all hold hands in a circle so they are all connected. The facilitator then leads a group healing meditation saying something like:

Script for Closing Group Healing Meditation

Here we all are now sitting together hands in hands, and each in contact with one of these special stones. Perhaps these are also mystical and mythical and mysterious stones, healing stones. They are something really solid to base life and change on, are they not? And, each one now has within it all of those interesting and powerful and wonderful ways of being and functioning that you have put into them, fused and part of them. And, somehow, somehow, just holding them in your hand and being in contact with each other makes this all a bit more real and powerful. Yes.

And, we are together now, hand in hand, heart to heart, mind to mind, and spirit to spirt. Sharing in this giving and receiving. So many wonderful gifts. We can just thank each other now, gently squeeze each other's hand, and just return here and now back to this room. Thank you for your sharing and your gifts to each of us. You each have your own stone now to keep and to hold.

Commentary

The closing healing meditation is needed to concretize and make real this sharing experience. This procedure can be repeated for any of the other concerns listed above, and also for any special concern raised by a group member.

25.5 Other Activities for Palliative Care Patients

In this section are presented a number of other activities for palliative care patients.

A. Videotaping

When people are nearing the end of their life and they know this either via a six-month prognosis that entitles them to enter a hospice program or a chronic disease or a debilitating and limiting one like ALS, it is useful to do something that validates their life. Most people do not prepare their own obituaries or plan their own celebration of life memorial services. An excellent way to validate their life is to make a video of them, generally a one- or two-hour one of them talking about their life. The interviewer needs to lead them through their life by asking questions. (If the palliative care patient is present with a spouse, then s/he is included in the interview and talks about her/his life. The couple also talks about their life together.) I have made many such recordings of people who almost all state at the outset that they can only think of a few things to talk about, and then easily go on and on. The very talking about their lives knowing that they are making a lasting record that can be passed on to family and friends is validating. It is therefore highly recommended that palliative care programs either arrange for such recordings or encourage their patients to do so. Older children or grandchildren can also do this.

B. Memoirs

Patients can also be encouraged to write their memoirs or record them. This is also a validation of life experience for people can vividly recall the important parts of their lives and what they have done or where they have traveled.

C. Pets, Stuffed Animals, and Special Belongings

Many people have pets who provide companionship and comfort. One friend who was quite old and knew that he would probably not live more than one year made a conscious choice with his wife to obtain a cat. He died not long ago, the cat sat on his hospice supplied bed in his living room, and his wife now enjoys having the cat as a companion. Many nursing homes have resident dogs or cats or volunteers bringing visiting dogs. I have also noticed in a local nursing home that many of the residents have stuffed animals. Some residents have plants that they can still tend. And, most are encouraged to have special pictures or even furniture or bed spreads or clothing in their rooms. All of these things need to be mentioned to palliative care patients.

D. Music

In addition to the ubiquitous TV sets in medical facilities some consideration also needs to be given to CD players and radios with or without head phones.

25.6 Hypnosis for Palliative Care and Pain Control

Considering my working definition for hypnosis, which is any time your attention is so focused on something that the work around you recedes, it is evident that in addition to guided imagery some of the other things discussed in this chapter also involve patients being in some level of trance. (Chapter 3 discusses using hypnosis for preparation for surgery.) In this section the use of hypnosis for pain control is discussed. Please note that there is an extensive literature on this subject going back to Esdaille's remarkable operations in India using hypnosis as the only anesthetic (1846, 1902). Also, see Barber and Adrian (1982) and Barber (1996).

The common rating scale for pain is to ask the patient to rate it on a scale of 0 to 10, where 0 is no pain at all and 10 it the most intense pain they can think of or have experienced. A second scale is useful and it is to rate how much the pain *bothers* them from 0 to 10, where 0 is no bother at all and 10 is extremely bothersome. Suggesting that in-between numbers like 3.4 and 7.8 can be used provides additional information. The use of *both* scales is important since some pains are more bothersome than others, and vice versa.

Pain is a warning signal and has a protective effect in allowing painful areas to be rested and given time to heal. Kay Thompson (1976) wrote about "appropriate pain" as follows, "When everything that can be done, and should be done, has been done, there is no longer any reason for pain. You can be pleasantly surprised how very comfortable it will be as long as normal healing is progressing."

Here, briefly discussed, are six methods using hypnosis for pain control.

1   *Distraction*—This is simply thinking of something else (and ignoring the pain). The suggestion is to think of being somewhere and at some time when you were really feeling comfortable. Have the patient think about being there, and then and have them practice triggering this experience with a normal movement like bringing two fingers together any time this is needed. (Milton Erickson distracted a woman who had cancer pain by saying to her, "Now tell me, Madam, if you saw a lean, hungry tiger in the next room, slowly walking into the room and eyeing you hungrily and licking its chops, how much pain would you feel?" She said the pain would leave her under those circumstances, and it did!)
2   *Dissociation*—Milton Erickson told another cancer patient that in his dreams he could be in a car or a boat or in the other room. Since his body was having the pain right here, why not feel himself somewhere else, just as he did in his dreams. This is like drifting out of your body and observing it from a distance, i.e., you were dissociated from it.

3 *Time Distortion*—Many pains like those in childbirth and some cancers (and other cases) are periodic. Patients can be taught to look at an imagined clock with hour, minute and second hands. They are then to imagine that in between the pains the clock slows down, and that during the pain the second and minute hands speed up. This imagery is then practiced. (We have all had the experience of time "dragging" or going very fast. Or, it's like being so deeply engaged in reading or a movie or a concert and then being surprised how much time has passed!)

4 *Nerve Switch*—Pain is transmitted from its bodily location to the brain via nerves. You can have your patient imagine that there is an on/off switch in the sensory nerve, and then practice turning off that switch (just like turning off a light).

5 *Glove Anesthesia*—One way is to have the person imagine being a child playing in the snow without gloves. Soon the hands get so cold that all feeling leaves them. Then, have them imagine moving one of those "frozen" hands to wherever in the body they are experiencing pain and holding it in that area. The numbness in the hand is then transmitted to that part of the body. This is practiced. Another way of doing this is having the person put a hand in a glass of ice water until it becomes numb (or imagining doing this) and then moving that to the painful location.

6 *Anticipated Pain and Remembered Pain*—A patient can be taught *amnesia* for their pain so that they do not look forward *or* back to the pains. "There are so many things that we can remember and forget and forgot to remember forgetting what it was that we remembered when we forgot to remember, are there not?" [This confusing statement induces the amnesia.]

Of course, the psychologist (or other health professional) who uses hypnosis for pain control needs to needs to be experienced in using hypnosis. (Special training and practice may be needed.)

25.7 Closing Comments

Section 15.3 is about physical health and coping skills. Since a large part of palliative care involves coping skills, they are important to know (but will not be repeated here). It is wonderful that we live at a time when palliative care has become a standard medical practice.

Note

1 This information is from http://reportcard.capc.org. A 2011 poll indicated that 95% of respondents agreed that it was important that patients with serious illness and their families be educated about palliative care.

26 Extraordinary Sessions¹

an ember glows
shadows dance on its surface
a flame hurtles out

A number of years ago at a public lecture I heard Alan Arkin tell about some of his experiences as an actor. A question from the audience requesting him to tell us about his best performance elicited an interesting story. Basically, he told us, professional actors are professionals and their performances essentially show us how well they have learned their craft. He is a good actor, and he was proud of the various roles he played in film, on TV, and on the stage. Arkin then told us that, in his experience, most actors rarely had that once-in-a-lifetime performance where they know, really know inside themselves, that they have given an extraordinary performance. The audience knows that they have transcended the boundary of routine excellence, and have attained a greatness—however transient—of a kind of immortality in their profession. These unique performances become the subject of legend: "Do you remember the night when XXX did that incredible Hamlet?" Arkin stated that he had had this particular experience on a few rare occasions, although he would not share those times with us. This, apparently, was too personal for him.

In this chapter I am going to expand on this theme with some personal examples related to acting and being a therapist, some literature examples, and then invite you to ponder on what this means to you and the profession of psychotherapy, and other professions.

Over the years I have acted and directed in community theater. About 30-plus years ago I had the supporting role of Boraccio in Shakespeare's *Much Ado About Nothing*. The play was put on in the summer in the outdoor amphitheater of Antioch College, and was directed by the well-known director Meredith Dallas (Dal). There were performances over two long weekends. As is usual, we had a "brush-up" rehearsal between the weekends. Boraccio is a drunkard and a braggart. I had one long speech that I struggled with—I hunted for the phrasing that made the meaning of Shakespeare's words clearly understandable. Dal insisted that we deliver the lines so that the audience heard distinctly every one of Shakespeare's words. In effect, he said that we could sacrifice "acting" to understanding, hoping that somehow the play would triumph through the playwright's words.

In my big scene in the brush-up I sat at the edge of a platform at center stage and delivered my one long speech. I have little memory of delivering that speech. When I finished, the entire cast and crew gave me a standing ovation. What happened? This was one of those Alan Arkin times. "Something" just came over me—rather, it took me over—and I went on to give the performance of my life. In *Star Wars* terms you might say that the "Force" was with me. It was a transcendental and transformational experience, for in retrospect I became another person, a separate persona, for that brief period of time. I was certain I was in some kind of trance state, watching and listening to myself as if from another world. Then it was over, and I "woke up" to the applause of my colleagues, being as startled as clients sometimes are when they are aroused from a hypnotic state. The show went on. Perhaps it is needless to say that in the following nights I did my usual capable acting, yet it was "usual" and "normal" without any repetition of the earlier exceptional speech. By some unfathomable prescience, the publicity photo for the play was of me in an earlier rehearsal doing that particular speech! As an aside, consider that this photo should have had the lead actors in it rather than me! I had my magic moment on the stage.

During the course of my four-plus decades as a counselor I have experienced this phenomenon several times with clients. There have been sessions where I "woke up" at the end knowing that I had exceeded my normal level of professionalism, and had achieved a special breakthrough with that client that proved to be lasting and unique. I said all the right things in the right way and with the right rapport for something special to occur. On some of those occasions the clients appeared to be surprised and even startled at what had happened to them. It is not unusual for me to be in some level of trance myself during sessions, although I always keep my eyes open and am intensely focused on the client and his/her reactions. (Milton Erickson has written that he was almost invariably in a trance state when working with clients, and would write his clinical notes afterwards in an automatic writing fashion.) I know that on those occasions I was working at the limits of my skills, mostly unconsciously, but with sufficient awareness to *consciously* guide the process. This may seem paradoxical, yet there is a conscious component to the unconscious mind.

Are there ways to increase the likelihood of working in this manner? Certainly, we can carefully observe some masters in the field like Milton H. Erickson, Ernest L. Rossi, Joseph Barber, and Steve Gilligan to get clues. In my observation of sessions carried out by these psychotherapists I have frequently had the sensation that not only were they in trance, but that they were operating from what we might call another plane of existence. I suspect that the more skilled and experienced you are, the greater the probability that this will happen to you on occasion.

Perhaps the most extraordinary example of this was a demonstration by Ernest L. Rossi, Ph.D., at the Erickson Congress in Phoenix in 1992. Before I write more about that, let me point out that the session so affected Rossi that he scrapped his prepared keynote speech for the following day, and essentially spoke about this demonstration. Rossi has written about this in detail in two chapters of his book on the psychobiology of gene expression (Rossi, 2002).[2] He seeded the kind of volunteer he wanted with the following opening remarks (Rossi, 2002, p. 302):

> For most of us, hypnosis is really about healing ... is it not? So I would like to ask if there is anyone in the audience this afternoon who is really in *an acute state of distress? Chronic distress, physical, mental, pain?* Someone who really has got *an issue that they feel they can do some effective work with this afternoon?* So, this is not merely a demonstration, this is the real thing! [emphases in original]

His volunteer was a young woman who had rheumatoid arthritis, particularly in her hands, for the last ten years. Rossi devoted almost one hundred pages of his book to a detailed analysis of the transcript, with special attention to his theories connecting gene expression and neurogenesis to hypnosis and psychotherapy. In line with the thesis of this paper, I would like to offer a different interpretation.

Rossi is a master of reading body language and also a master of what I call "minimalism." (By " minimalism" I mean that he uses the absolute minimum of words to assist a client in doing her own work.) His *expectation* is that the client will do meaningful work in this session. After eliciting information about her condition, he asks her, " Celeste, tell me just where you are experiencing it ...," followed shortly thereafter with, "Stay with that ache for a moment Celeste and let's see what happens with it when you focus on it now." Then, he just lets her experience her own sensations while he guides her with brief comments to continue to explore what is happening to those sensations. Rossi also uses *long pauses* to allow the client to do her inner work. A good example of this (Rossi, 2002, p. 316) is: "[long pause] That's right, *the courage to really go with it,* Celeste, and *occasionally saying a few words or a sentence ... only what I need to hear* [pause] *to help you further.* [long pause]" Celeste had entered into a trance earlier when she focused inwardly. Although one part of Rossi's mind was certainly aware that he was doing a demonstration before perhaps one thousand people and had a time limit for this work, he was also in a mutual trance state with Celeste, where the two of them were intensely concentrating—she on her internal work, and he on her. At the end of this session (which really needs to be studied in detail), these are the final comments (Rossi, 2002, p. 390):

> [Celeste extended both hands forward and straight in an open gesture, as if to show the audience how well she was.] How does that look to you, the audience?
>
> [There is loud, extended clapping from the audience, while Celeste smiles with delight and I clap my hands and gaze at her with appreciation. I then stand up, still clapping, and inviting Celeste to stand with her hands upward in triumph.]
>
> Whoa! Whoa! Whoa!

Those of us in the audience, Celeste, and Rossi had all shared in this miraculous hour of theatre, of witnessing two human beings who were in such intimate rapport that the world around them had receded, and both trans-formations and *trance*-formations have occurred. It was evident to everyone, especially the two key actors, that they had all participated in something extraordinary, something beyond the expectation of competence. Rossi (2002, p. 352) comments earlier, "However, I really don't know what is happening at this moment. The simple truth is that most therapists and patients are blind to what is really important most of the time on an implicit level." Rossi is so skilled at engaging clients at the deepest levels of interpersonal contact via his minimalism, that it is not surprising that I have observed him doing similar work at other conferences.

In an attempt to clarify what I have been describing, I return to my own evolution as a therapist as a possible way of enhancing the likelihood of these special occurrences. In recent times I have grown into a style that I call "chatting," something I have discussed earlier in this book. What is the connection between this way of functioning and Arkin's talk? For me, the connection is that the chatting style seems to make it more probable that I will have one of those exceptional sessions *in toto*, or in part. There is so much more involvement, person-to-person, that there is little room for being overly consciously directive and thinking about interventions. My conscious concentration on the client and what he/she is saying and doing means that I am in some level of trance where the focus of my trance is the client and not my cognitive thinking and analyzing. Also, as an example, with all of the conscious design in Erickson's work with clients, and all of the careful seeding that he did, the *intensity* of his focus on the client can be considered to be the primary instrument of his rapport and change work.

This is obviously a personal matter, and I do not know how what I have written here will translate into the way others practice. I am suggesting to you, the reader, that this style of involvement has advantages that can be product-ively explored.

Notes

1 After I wrote this essay, I shared it with my friend and colleague Michael F. Hoyt. We decided it would be a good idea for a book featuring many people we would invite to share similar experiences. In researching this topic we found that there was a literature on this subject, and also one book. We therefore abandoned the project. I decided when I got to editing the last part of this book that the essay (edited for this book) would be a good last full chapter.

2 A videotape of this session is available for health professionals from the Milton H. Erickson Foundation, 3606 North 24th Street, Phoenix, AZ 85016 as IC-92-D-V9.

27 Some Ending Thoughts and Comments

late afternoon sun
stretches shadows silently
fragile fairy light

This book is deliberately personal. That is, I have written about a whole bunch of things that have become special to me in the practice of the very brief therapy that is anchored in many areas I have studied, and is centered around the uses of hypnosis, which are strongly influenced by my studies of Milton Erickson and his work. At one point in my life when I was writing my biography of Erickson in play form I was totally immersed in his work and writings and the recordings of him in action. During that time I was blessed and fortunate to have the support and help of two of his daughters—Roxanna Erickson Klein and the late Betty Alice Erickson. When I am that immersed in a writing project it is like being in a waking conscious trance state. It is also the case that I am frequently "transcribing" from memory bits and pieces I have thought about during wakeful times at night, and lying in bed in the morning. Those are wonderful and cherished times.

I am writing this section before I go back into a final editing mode. This is a new style for me, and is the first book I have written that incorporates many case studies.[1] Also, I am soon to be 89 years old and this is a time when thoughts of mortality sneak in more frequently, especially when I am finding the loneliness that my brother Ralph experienced as he aged. Ralph died at the end of March 2019 in his 100th year of life, and often told me that there was only one friend from his earlier years who was still alive. My oldest and closest friend from high school died two years ago, and in recent months more than five friends here in Yellow Springs have died. So, I continue to write and work out in the weight room at the university and hike and go to movies and theater and read books and marvel that spring has once more appeared with all of its greenery. People and Nature are what it is all about, isn't it?

At this point I am going to indulge in printing a group of my three-line poems that appeared in the *Yellow Springs News* (May 16, 2019 issue).[2] They are preceded by the following comments I submitted with the poems.

Please find below four of my three-line poems for the *YS News*. I was first inspired to write in this style when I read Haiku with its 5/7/5 syllable format and concise descriptions. I know that my three-line poems are not Haiku and certainly my poems frequently have a different syllable count. My goal has been to capture an image, emotion, idea, person or moment in a few words. I know that readers unconsciously "speak" the lines of poetry when they read them. So, another goal was to add

sonority to the poems.

almost frozen stream
air bubbles rippling under ice
quiet crystals

snowflakes
swiftly swirling and soaring
settle into white

the crinkle of ice
falling from weighted branches
sprinkling bright on snow

in weary winter
bare branches scratch skyward
a lone leaf flutters

THANK YOU

Notes

1 As I have written earlier in this book, almost all of the case studies are "reconstructions" based on brief case notes and my usual style of working with clients.
2 Other poems have appeared throughout this book including the opening of each chapter.

Appendix A: Ruminations on Turning 88[1]

the old man is gone
his hopes and dreams quietly
passing in the night

On June 22 of the year 2019 I turned 88, that is, I entered the 89th year of my life. Having completed a number of other activities, I decided for several reasons to write these ruminations at this time. In part this is inspired by my friend John Bett's memoirs in four parts that we have been privileged to read. He was born in Scotland, and went to school there before enrolling at the Illinois Institute of Technology in Chicago in its Ph.D. program in chemistry. I was a young faculty member in the department at that time and we were roughly the same age. We became fast friends, and he was our best man when Charlotte and I married in 1960. (We still keep in touch with him and his wife, Emily.) I now have in mind that sometime in the near future I will write a full set of memoirs.

A few months ago something happened when I was swimming in the outdoor pool in Yellow Springs. In recent years I have only been swimming in the summer. When I started as a faculty member in the chemistry department at Wright State University in 1966 there was a group of faculty members who would swim regularly at the YMCA pool in nearby Fairborn. After a while, the university had its own swimming pool, and I swam there for quite a few years. (Now I work out regularly in the university weight room and do other exercises.)

Once upon a time I could actually swim the entire length of the pool (25 yards then) under water (later, this became swimming the width of the pool under water). Also, at that time in the 15 minutes that youngsters were kicked out of the pool in a "rest" period I could also swim 18 lengths (one-fourth of a mile) during that time. As I have aged the number of laps has slowly declined until this past summer they were mostly in the 8–12 range (although I did swim the 18 lengths once, taking more than 15 minutes). However, the one thing I have always been proud of is that I could swim the entire first length (now 25 meters) on one breath, and I was able to do that most of the time. This all stopped about three months ago when after I had done that and was continuing to do some leisurely laps that I had to stop as I was feeling light-headed and dizzy. At that time I wondered if this was a stroke, but I managed to carefully get out of the pool, take a brief shower, and drive home. I told Charlotte about this and slowly recuperated—the light-headedness lasted for a moderately long time. We talked about this and basically decided that I had "overdone" the swimming and that this was a signal that something had to change in my "macho" way of swimming. As the end of the swimming season was approaching and we had some foul weather to boot, I did not get to swim again—if I had returned to the pool I would have wisely turned to swimming more leisurely! One thing I will especially miss is swimming the last two lengths on my back and leisurely looking at the clouds in the sky. So, the incident described in this paragraph is the inspiration for these ruminations.

Last year and this year Charlotte and I had tentatively planned on a trip to Europe at the end of the summer. When time ran away with us we thought we would do some local traveling. We ended up doing neither, although we made some trips in the spring and in June for family events. I did go to New York at the end of March to attend my brother Ralph's funeral—he died towards the end of his one hundredth year, and after making a medical decision about never walking again (he broke his hip) or risking an operation. So, all of the above is leading to decisions to slow down and change your life style.

I had decided earlier in the year to not continue doing the chemistry demonstration shows for middle and high school students that I had done for over 40 years. My longtime partner in doing those shows, John Fortman, had not been with me for over two years due to his health. For perhaps 30 years my volunteer work was being the facilitator for a semi-monthly support group for caregivers (the Charlie Brown group), and those who have or had life-challenging diseases. This group was modeled on Bernie Siegel's Exceptional Cancer Patient (ECaP) groups. Earlier this year the attendance at our meetings at the Senior Center in Yellow Springs kept declining to the point where there was only me and one or two other people. I put a reminder of the availability of this group in the local newspaper and there were no new attendees. It appeared to me and the few people attending that it was now time to close this group down and I did so.

Several months or so ago I also withdrew from a commitment to be one of the speakers at a hypnosis training group in Mexico. I was the only American who was repeatedly invited back to their annual meetings, got to know and love many of the people in the group, and felt close to them. I was scheduled to be one of the main speakers at their meeting in Huatulco (Oaxaca province in southernmost Mexico). We worked out a complicated way for me to travel back and forth to the meeting that I (and they) thought would be the least wearing on me. Two things decided me to cancel: when I looked at the new itinerary I realized that the transit time on the day I was traveling was going to be of the order of 12–14 hours with two significant stopovers and being on three planes. I would leave on a morning flight from Columbus, OH, and arrive in Huatulco late in the evening. The second item was a health issue with Charlotte that has continued to be unresolved and has involved a number of tests and doctors. I just needed to be here to be with her. I also do all of the out-of-area driving now, and all driving to doctors and tests. I miss my Mexican friends and colleagues and regret having to disappoint them. (My Mexican friends did arrange for me to do a teleconference of one of my intended workshops, and that went well.) So, all of this has led me to thinking about what I am capable of now, and what I want to do with the rest of my life.

Another hallmark change is that this coming December (2019) will be the last of the Erickson conferences on hypnosis and psychotherapy. I have been on the faculty of many of these conferences in the past, and will be doing a number of presentations at this one. In addition to learning a great deal at these meetings, they were always an opportunity to spend time with colleagues I had come to know over the years, and who became part of my extended family.

This reconsideration of what is really important in life and how I have functioned in the past has been influenced by a historian and social scientist named Lewis Mumford and his work. I want to share that with my readers now. In searching the web for his work and looking at the extensive write-up of his contributions in Wikipedia I did not find a reference to what I recall he described as the "industrial imperative." My memory told me that what he wrote was, "If it is possible, it has to be done." And, in his writings, he stated that this is what has driven civilization, especially Western civilization, since the industrial revolution in the nineteenth century. The closest I have come to this recalled definition in the web is, *"technology imperative.* The concept that new technologies are inevitable and essential and that they must be developed and accepted for the good of society." So, I go back to: "If it is possible, it has to be done," and these ruminations are an exploration of that imperative in my life. (It may also be—or have been—the driving force in the lives of many readers of this piece.)

So, how far back in my life am I going to go to find examples of that "imperative?" I was not a daring or adventurous person in my childhood and teens. I was a bit on the timid side, and socially inept. In fact, I was quite awkward about girls although I thought about them a lot in my teens. I did have two significant girlfriends in my high school days. They were first Gloria G. and later Marilyn S. (I also dated Marilyn through my college days.) To refresh my memory, I just got out my high school year book. Although my memory has me as not being very outgoing or sociable, in thumbing through that yearbook I just found that almost everyone (maybe 90%) of my classmates wrote something in it next to their photos. Wow!

Of my classmates there were only two that I kept up with in the sense that we were in touch until the end of their lives. The first was Victor Bloom who ended up getting a medical degree, and then became a psychoanalyst. We exchanged many emails over a fairly long period of time. He never believed my comments about how I worked as a brief therapist (and then a single-session one), and I could never understand how he could be professionally ethical and see clients for five to ten years. He lived in Grosse Point, MI, and the last time I saw him was in Ann Arbor where his son drove him to meet up with me for lunch on one of my trips there to spend time with my friend and colleague Howard Fink. We ate at Zingerman's Deli and spent an amiable time together. (Bloom died about three years ago.) Perhaps my closet and oldest friend was George Forrester. We both went to the Bronx High School of Science and The City College of CCNY. I majored in chemistry. George was expected by his parents to be a dentist (mine expected me to be a medical doctor). George joined Dramsoc, the college theater group, met his future wife, Gilda, there, and was thoroughly captivated by the theater. After gradu-ation, he and Gilda married, followed by two years in the army where he did theater work. Eventually, George became a Professor of Theater at San Jose State College, and an acknowledged actor and director. George died about two years ago, and I continue to keep in touch with Gilda. To each other we were extended family, and Charlotte and I visited with them whenever we visited our family in Folsom. When we were together it was always as if we lived down the street from each other and picked up our conversation in that mode. (I hope that whoever reads this has similar "relatives.")

Going back to my high school year book I found that I wrote my own "tribute" to myself in the following poem, which was signed "George Freeman," which was a pseudonym I used for a while when I was a teenager (I do not recall now why I did that!):

> To a fellow:
> Who I am sure
> Will find the cancer cure,
> Will climb the highest mountain,
> Will for eternal youth a fountain
> Find in the depths of the jungle,
> Will never a hard task bungle,
> "Great men never feel great,
> small men never feel small"
> This my friend can relate,
> For you see, he's been them all.
> What holds the future?
> A forceps or suture?
> We will be a writer

Or maybe a fighter.
My prediction is that he will be,
A man who DOES & wants to SEE.

As I write this, I am looking back to the predictions I made 70 years ago. No cancer cure, no medical degree, no mountaineering (lots of hiking, though, and in many high places). Over the years I have written many plays and much poetry, about 100 each of chemical education papers and chemical research ones, a few chemistry books, and ten books related to the field of psychotherapy. So, much to look back on.

One of the things that has troubled me for a long time is a sense that somehow I have sneaked through life doing and accomplishing many things without feeling that I really did them or was competent enough to do them. I admired others for being smarter than I was and more knowledgeable, and who found it easier to be social and interact with people. That is, I felt like an impostor who somehow really did not deserve to be where I was professionally as a chemistry professor or as a therapist. My friend Michael Hoyt wrote to me that this was a common phenomenon that had been recognized and written about in the literature for a long time. Also, it was fairly common. It is called the "Impostor Syndrome" or IS. The earliest description of it I found was a paper published in 1978. Two recent books are cited in the footnote,[2] but the Wikipedia entry on it is excellent. Its introduction states:

> Impostor syndrome (also known as impostor phenomenon, impostorism, fraud syndrome or the impostor experience) is a psychological pattern in which an individual doubts their accomplishments and has a persistent internalized fear of being exposed as a "fraud." Despite external evidence of their competence, those experiencing this phenomenon remain convinced that they are frauds, and do not deserve all they have achieved. Individuals with impostorism incorrectly attribute their success to luck, or as a result of deceiving others into thinking they are more intelligent than they perceive themselves to be.

The article further states, "It has been estimated that nearly 70 per cent of individuals will experience signs and symptoms of the impostor phenomenon at last once in their life." Also, somewhere I read that most people with IS believe that this is a rare thing that has only happened to them! I certainly had no idea of its prevalence.

So, I will tell one personal story about this, and also how I believe people may get over it. A long time ago when I was an assistant professor in the chemistry department at the Illinois Institute of Technology in Chicago, I overheard two colleagues say that they really admired me. I did not overhear what it was about which I was being admired! I was quite surprised to hear this since I thought that both of these colleagues were much smarter than me and were better chemists. So, this puzzled me. It is now over 60 years since I heard that. I do know that I was aware of my abilities and capabilities in chemistry since I decided at that time to devote my chemistry career to two areas: chemical education since I was very interested in effective teaching; and the second was in doing the very best experimental research. I felt that I did not have the background in theory and mathematics or the ability to do abstract and theoretical work, but I was very good at measuring phenomena. So, that is what I did, and earned a reputation in both areas, even though doubts persisted. It is characteristic of IS people that they believe the statement at the end of the indented quote above.

My solution to IS-ism is to do two things. The first is to just recognize that in all areas that there are people who are more skilled, smarter, and talented than just about anybody in their fields. So be it. I believe that I excelled in two areas of chemistry[3] and that is really enough, is it not? The second is to just be aware (and accept!) that I have made contributions in chemistry and psychotherapy that others in those fields have recognized. It is enough, is it not, to simply do the best you can?

Some Concluding Thoughts

Looking back over my life I am content now at what I have done, and also that on the way I have made many friends and helped many people. There is also much satisfaction in being a father and grandfather and father-in-law. As indicated above, I am not sure how all of these offspring have turned out so well, and am not going to dwell on that—just enjoy it! So, at this time I have pulled back from many endeavors, and added one, which is a monthly master class for psychotherapists. My small primarily single-session therapy practice appears to be working, too. The future most likely holds less traveling, perhaps an attempt at writing my memoirs, as much time with family and friends as is feasible, and hopefully a few surprises.

Notes

1   This essay written on 10/20/19.
2   Clance, P. R. (1985). Hillman, H. (2013).
3   The first is in the number of publications I have in chemical education and a number of innovations I made in that field. The second is that in chemistry research the work that I and my research colleagues did on the high precision solubility of gases in water will probably never be exceeded. (We attained a precision of ca. 0.02% in that work.) Also, many of my research papers (with colleagues) involving physical chemical measurements were of high precision.

Appendix B: End-of-Life Issues

mourning sun
glowing on the gravestone
a flower wilts

B.I Introduction

I have heard Bernie Siegel do a number of presentations, and he almost always said sometime, "No one gets out of this world alive."[1] So, we will all die. The questions then are when, how, what we do between now and then, and how we anticipate we will feel and change as our time of death gets closer. We can make plans for our death at any age. When we are young that time is off somewhere in the distant future. When I was young I rarely thought about this and I believe I felt then that I was kind of immortal. Soon to be 89 I do think more about my own death, yet it still seems to be unreal.

A while back I reviewed Irvin D. Yalom's book (2008, 2009) entitled, *Staring at the Sun. Overcoming the Terror of Death.* In this remarkable book, Yalom writes about, "what I have learned about overcoming the terror of death from my own experience, my work with patients, and the thoughts of those writers who have informed my own work." I learned much from reading his book and consider the following quotations as being excellent introductory material.

- My personal and clinical work have taught me that anxiety about dying waxes and wanes throughout the life cycle. [Children note the glimmerings of mortality surrounding them, and the fear of death appears to go underground from about six to puberty.] (p. 3)
- It's not easy to live every moment wholly aware of death. It's like trying to stare the sun in the face: you can stand only so much of it. Because we cannot live frozen in fear, we generate methods to soften death's terror. ... Some people—supremely confident in their immunity—live heroically, often without regard for others or for their own safety. ... Death anxiety

is the mother of all religions, which, in one way or another, attempt to temper the anguish of our finitude. (p. 5)

- I believe that we should confront death as we confront other fears. We should contemplate our ultimate end, familiarize ourselves with it, dissect and analyze it, reason with it, and discard terrifying childhood death distortions. ... Let's not conclude that death is too painful to bear, that the thought will destroy us, that transiency must be denied lest the truth render life meaningless. Such denial always exacts a price ... Anxiety will always accompany our confrontation with death. (p. 276)

- I do not intend this to be a solemn book. Instead, it is my hope that by grasping, really grasping, our human condition—our finiteness, our brief time in the light—we will come not only to savor the preciousness of each moment and the pleasure of sheer being but to increase our compassion for ourselves and all other human beings. (p. 277) [from the Afterword]

To quote from my review,

> Perhaps the most important idea in the book is that of *rippling* (chapter 4). This refers to the idea that each of us creates, usually without conscious intent or knowledge, "... concentric circles of influence that may affect others for years, even generations." (p. 83) That is, we live on in others, and these ripples flow on and on and ...

In Chapter 6 of his book Yalom shares his own fear of death. And, he shares this in the last lines of a poem he wrote a long time ago:

> till stone is laid on stone
> and though none can hear
> and none can see
> each sobs softly: remember me, remember me

The longest chapter in his book (7) is all about advice for therapists in addressing death anxiety in their clients and themselves. It is full of useful ideas.

This chapter briefly covers many topics associated with end-of-life issues, and it ends with an annotated list of references. My wife and I attended the Dying With Dignity world meeting in Chicago in September 2015. We learned a great deal there, and much of it is in this chapter. I joined an ad hoc committee to explore finding a better phrase for describing this movement and what it is about. We worked for almost one year, and explored many phrases and words. Part of the motivation for this was to get away from the word "suicide," which, of course, is an action of "dying with dignity." A good descriptive is "self-deliverance." At the end of our studies we decided to keep "dying with dignity" for organizations and meetings. My preferred phrase, which covers all of the aspects about this *for me* is:

Dying with Dignity, Choice, Control, Comfort, and Companionship

B.2 Advanced Directives

Advanced directives are basically legal documents which you can fill out describing what your wishes are for the end of your life. They are of two types:

1 *Living Will*: This spells out the types of medical treatments you want at the end of your life if you are unable to speak for yourself. It tells medical professionals your wishes regarding specific treatments such as medical ventilation or tube feeding.
2 *Health Care Power of Attorney* (or Durable Power of Attorney for Health): This document appoints someone to make health care decisions on your behalf when you cannot communicate on your own. This covers a range of medical treatments which you specify.

There are two really important caveats here: the first is that these become effective when you can no longer communicate your own wishes; and the second is that each state in the U.S. has its own set of these documents. You should be able to obtain these forms and instructions for free from your state. When you have filled them out you need witnesses when you sign, and you may also require notarization. (DNR or do not resuscitate orders and POLST and MOLST physician orders differ by state, and will be discussed separately below.) A really important thing about any of these advance directives is to be sure that you have discussed them with your children (and your specified agent) and that they are on board with your intentions. If any of them are not, then you definitely need to only use the ones who are willing to go along with your wishes in your advanced directives.

A. Living Will

This form provides four choices for you to select under the two headings of: "If I am in a terminal condition" and "If I am in a permanently unconscious state." These four choices are: (1) Administer no life-sustaining treatment, including CPR and artificially or technologically supplied nutrition or hydration; (2) Withdraw such treatment, including CPR, if such treatment has started; (3) Issue a DNR order; and (4) Permit me to die naturally and take no action to postpone my death, providing me with only that care necessary to make me comfortable and to relieve my pain.

B. Health Care Power of Attorney

The guidance to the named agent (there can be up to two alternate agents specified) is:

> My agent will make health care decisions for me based on the instructions that I give in this document and on my wishes otherwise known to my agent. If my agent believes that my wishes as made known to my agent conflict with what is in this document, this document will control. If my wishes are unclear or unknown, my agent will make health care decisions in my best interests. My agent will determine my best interests after considering the benefits, the burdens, and the risks that might result from a given decision. If no agent is available, this document will guide decisions about my health care.

There are many legal choices you can make with respect to your end-of-life wishes. It is important to emphasize here the statements of your condition for these documents to be applied: "If I am in a terminal condition" and "If I am in a permanently unconscious state."

C. Do Not Resuscitate (DNR)

This authorizes a physician to write an order letting health care personnel know that a patient does not wish to be resuscitated in the event of cardiac arrest (no palpable pulse) or respiratory arrest (no spontaneous respirations or the absence of labored breathing). This is important in the case of "medical emergencies" such as those that occur when emergency personnel are called via a 911 call.

There are two generally options within the DNR Comfort Care Protocol and they are the DNR Comfort Care (DNRCC) Order and the DNR Comfort Care-Arrest (DNRCC-Arrest) Order. With a DNRCC Order, a person receives any care that eases pain and suffering, but no resuscitative measures to save or sustain life from the moment the order is signed by the physician. With a DNRCC-Arrest Order, a person receives standard medical care that may include some components of resuscitation until he or she experiences a cardiac or respiratory arrest. [FYI—I know some people who have had "DNR" tattooed to their chests to be sure that their requests in this regard will be honored, but this is not legally enforceable.]

D. POLST and MOLST

POLST stands for Physicians Order for Life-Sustaining Treatment, and MOLST stands for Medical Order for Life-Sustaining Treatment (the first—POLST—is more commonly used). Each state in the U.S.A. has its own laws regarding this, although they are similar. To be clear about options, there are two types of advance directives: living wills and health care proxy. Living wills identify types of treatment a patient wants or does not want if they are terminally ill or in a vegetative state and lack decision-making capacity. A health care proxy document identifies a surrogate to make decisions when the patient lacks decision-making capacity. [Please note that when there is a conflict as to which applies, the Living Will predominates.]

POLST is an actionable medical order. POLST is only for seriously ill patients for whom their health care professional (HCP) would not be surprised if they died in the next year. It is the culmination of a shared decision-making process between the patient and his/her HCP. In doing this the HCP identifies and discusses the patient's specific diagnosis, prognosis, and treatment options (including the benefits and burden of each). [The parenthetical comment is of particular importance when you are making these decisions, i.e., what will be the likely quality of your life after particular treatments?] The patient also shares his/her own values, beliefs, and goals. They work together on the final document, and the HCP signs it only after this. Two major items about a POLST are that there is a *one-year prognosis for life*, and that it is a *medical order* signed by a physician. The POLST document cannot appoint a surrogate decision-maker. Emergency personnel *must* follow this document. Finally, the POLST form is patient-centered, and honors the patient's moral and religious and personal beliefs and wishes.

E. Five Wishes

This is a useful group of wishes and are:

1. The Person I Want to Make Care Decisions for Me When I Can't.
2. The Kind of Medical Treatment I Want or Don't Want.
3. How Comfortable I Want to Be.
4. How I Want People to Treat Me.
5. What I Want My Loved Ones to Know.

You can find more details in the Five Wishes website (www.agingwithdignity/five-wishes).

F. MyDirectives

This is a free website www.mydirectives.com where you can store your end-of-life directions and wishes. The following are the categories of information you can store on this web site and which you can send to personal contacts and your health providers:

- My Current Medical Condition.
- My Medical Treatment Goals, Preferences, and Priorities.
- My Preferences in Special Circumstances.
- My End-of-Life Preferences.
- My Health Care Agent (with 1st and 2nd alternates).
- My Thoughts.
- Personal Contacts (who to contact).
- Health Care Providers (your medical providers).
- Insurance Providers.

You can fill in specific responses in each category and then send them to your personal contacts and health providers.

B.3 Dying With Dignity Organizations and Information

The founder of the dying with dignity movement was Derek Humphry. He organized many end-of-life support groups. He is the author of *Let Me Die Before I Wake, The Right to Die*, and *Freedom to Die*. His book, *Final Exit*, was on the *New York Times* bestseller list for 18 weeks and has been translated into 11 languages. He lives near Eugene, Oregon. (E-mail: derekhumphry@ starband.net.) (The full references for his books above will be found in the reference section under Humphry, D.) He continues to be the guiding inspirational force in the worldwide dying with dignity movement.

Humphry heads up the organization called ERGO (The Euthanasia Research & Guidance Organization). It was founded in 1993 to improve the quality of background research and information for hastening dying for persons who are terminally or hopelessly ill and wish to end their suffering. ERGO holds that voluntary euthanasia, assisted suicide, physician-assisted suicide, physician-assisted dying and self-deliverance, are all appropriate life endings depending on the individual medical and ethical circumstances. ERGO and FEN (see below) have supported research into self-deliverance methods described later in this chapter. Their website is: www.assistedsuicide. org, where you can find information and a bookstore. Richard Cote's book (2012) entitled *In Search of Gentle Death. The Fight for Your Right to Die with Dignity* is an excellent history of the movement. It is well-written and researched as Cote was a professional journalist.

A. Compassion & Choices

Their mission statement states, "We support, educate and advocate. Across the nation, we work to ensure healthcare providers honor and enable patients' decisions about their care." To make this vision a reality, Compassion &

Choices works nationwide in legislatures, Congress, courts, medical settings, and communities. Their website is: www.compassionandchoices.org. There are many local chapters around the U.S., and they are organized by state. They have been quite influential in the battles for establishing legal medical assistance in dying in the U.S. in states like Oregon, Washington, and California. Compassion & Choices also sponsor training and informational meetings. See their website (cited above).

B. Final Exit Network (FEN)

Wikipedia has the following about FEN:

> (FEN) is an American nonprofit right to die and pro-assisted suicide organization incorporated in Marietta, Georgia. It holds that mentally competent adults who suffer from terminal illnesses, intractable pain, or irreversible physical (though not necessarily terminal) conditions have a right to voluntarily end their lives and, if they desire, to seek assistance to that end. In cases deemed valid, the Final Exit Network arranges what it refers to as "self-deliverances." Typically, the network assigns two "exit guides" to a client and are present when they die, but the network insists that they do not take an active role in the "death event"; rather, their role is that of compassionate advisors and witnesses. Final Exit Network was founded in 2004 by former members of the Hemlock Society, including that organization's co-founders, Derek Humphry and Dr. Faye Girsh. It was named after Humphry's 1991 book of the same name. It is a member of the World Federation of Right to Die Societies.

This is an accurate description of FEN. (My wife and I have been members for a number of years.) In the above description you will note that the guides do not take an active role in self-deliverance. Assisting someone in committing suicide is illegal in the United States. Giving information about how a person may do this is not, and is implicit in the "free speech" guaranteed by the U.S. constitution. (Please note that there have been legal battles over this.) When someone requests an exit guide (volunteers who are thoroughly trained), the exit guide visits that person and goes through an extensive interview with them. This information is passed on to a group of three physicians who decide if the person meets all of the criteria for guidance. If the person is approved, then the exit guide meets with him/her and provides all of the necessary information for self-deliverance. The guide (and others) may be present at the time when the person uses the described method, but they cannot assist in any way. (Methods of self-deliverance are discussed later in this chapter.) The FEN service is free and is supported by donations. Their website is: www.finalexitnetwork.org. Please note that both FEN and Compassion & Choices provide free lecturers.

C. World Federation of Right to Die Societies (WFRtDS)

The World Federation (www.worldrtd.net), founded in 1980, consists of 51 right to die organizations from 26 countries. The Federation provides an international link for organizations working to secure or protect the rights of individuals to self-determination at the end of their lives. Their free news-letter (sign up online) provides up-to-date information about their annual conferences, all of their member organizations, and useful papers and articles. (My wife and I attended one of their meetings.)

D. Death Cafés

Their website (www.deathcafe.com) describes their organization as:

> At a Death Café people, often strangers, gather to eat cake, drink tea and discuss death. Our objective is "to increase awareness of death with a view to helping people make the most of their (finite) lives." A Death Café is a group directed discussion of death with no agenda, objectives or themes. It is a dis-cussion group rather than a grief support or counselling session. Our Death Cafés are always offered: (a) On a not for profit basis; (b) In an accessible, respectful and confidential space; (c) With no intention of leading people to any conclusion, product or course of action; and (d) Alongside refreshing drinks and nourishing food—and cake!

Their website contains more information about locations of Death Cafés and how to organize and run them. A group discussion like this always needs an experienced facilitator. They do provide an opportunity to make people aware in a friendly setting of end-of-life issues.

E. Catholic Health Facilities

A guest speaker at an end-of-life group meeting I attended spoke on the sub-ject of advanced directives and Catholic health facilities. Every religion has its own standards and guidelines and beliefs and traditions related to death and dying. Funeral services vary greatly; for example, in Jewish tradition as one example, a person who has died needs to be buried within 24 hours if pos-sible. This means that funeral services and burial need to be arranged quickly. In many Jewish communities this is handled by a burial society to which they belong and which handles all of the arrangements.

The aforementioned speaker began his presentation with the information that in his home state of Washington that in 2013 that Catholic health facil-ities amounted to about 50% of those in the state. Some were owned outright by the church, and others were in mergers with other health facilities. The controlling factor is a decision by the U.S. Conference of Catholic Bishops. To quote from their ethical and religious directives (ERDS):

- "the directives promote and protect the truths of the Catholic faith as those truths are brought to bear on concrete issues in health care."
- Are subject to interpretation by local bishops.
- Apply to sponsors, trustees, administrators, chaplains, physicians, health care personnel, and patients or residents of Catholic institutions or services.

I believe patients need to be informed about these controlling factors in Catholic health facilities. Remember, you always have the right to be transferred to another hospital if any of the above items restrict your wants and needs. In the case of hospitals (or other facilities) that have merged with Catholic ones, you need to check the agreements between the Catholic administrators and the non-religious ones. For example, it may be possible to have an abortion or no artificial hydration and nutrition if so agreed upon.

F. Hospice Programs

The term "hospice" (from the same linguistic root as "hospitality") can be traced back to medieval times when it referred to a place of shelter and rest for weary or ill travelers on a long journey. The name was first applied to specialized care for dying patients by physician Dame Cicely Saunders, who began her work with the terminally ill in 1948 and eventually went on to create the first modern hospice—St. Christopher's Hospice—in a residential suburb of London.

There are several things to note about the functioning of hospice programs.

1 The patient can only be admitted to a hospice program if a medical doctor makes a prognosis that the patient is likely to die within six months.
2 Medicare funds hospice care for those who have this benefit.
3 Hospice care can be in the patient's home, a nursing home, or in a hospice facility.
4 In the beginning hospice programs were all non-profit. At present, most hospice programs are for profit.
5 Hospice programs are superb at controlling pain and other end-of-life difficulties.
6 Most hospice programs do palliative care and not just survival care.
7 When you are in a hospice program they provide all of the medical care that is needed including medications.

8 Hospice programs also provide pastoral care, economic guidance, grieving support and guidance, any needed social work, family support, and for those at home medical devices like hospital beds and oxygen.
9 Hospice programs do not do medical treatments to prolong life.

Many (probably most) hospices now also provide palliative care (see chapter 25).

G. Questions to Ask Before Tests and Procedures

Barbara Combs Lee who is the president of the organization Compassion & Choices has written a wonderful book and guide about death and dying in America (2019). In this section I present three series of questions regarding tests and treatments when you are old and your health may be deteriorating. Also, at the end of this section are the fascinating five things doctors know about end of life.

Before Consenting to a Test

1 What will the results of the test tell me/the doctor?
2 Will that information change the diagnosis, prognosis, or treatment options? How?
3 What are the burdens of the test in terms of pain, duration, and recovery time?
4 What can go wrong? What are the possible complications and/or what are the side effects?
5 What is the course of action without the test? (p. 110)

Before Consenting to a Treatment

1 What is the goal of this treatment, i.e., the expected outcome or response?
2 What proportion of people receiving this treatment achieve that goal? How often does it work for people in my situation?
3 If the goal is to prolong life, what is the expected increase in life expectancy? How many months or years?
4 What are the risks or side effects? How often do these occur?
5 How will this treatment affect the quality of my life? What is the frequency, duration, and recovery time after each treatment?
6 Is there a chance this treatment will make my condition worse?
7 Are there additional options beyond those you mentioned?
8 What will likely happen if I decline this treatment? (p. 113)

Medical Interventions You Can Decline or Stop in Order to Die Peacefully, with Medical Support

1   Renal dialysis.
2   Implanted defibrillator.
3   Ventilator, Bi-Pap or other breathing apparatus.
4   Cardiac pacemaker, for those with complete heart block.
5   Hi-tech cardiac support, such as an aortic pump.
6   Artificial feeding of any kind, via a nasal tube, tubes inserted in the stomach, or other method like hand feeding.
7   Antibiotics for any infection, especially pneumonia.
8   Insulin, to induce diabetic coma.
9   Medication for congestive heart failure, but only with excellent comfort care to treat symptoms. (p. 210)

Five Things Doctors Know about End of Life

1   Death is inevitable. Something will be the cause of death for every one of us.
2   We can and should expend great effort to remain healthy, but we should also put some effort into preparing to die well.
3   Medicine has never made a person immortal. All treatment plans will eventually "fail."
4   Keeping these truths in mind is the key to exercising discernment in one of life's most important decisions—when to turn away from futile therapies and focus completely on love, beauty, faith—the things that are the most important at the close of life.
5   Only the person dying can exercise this discernment, for it arises from their unique experience and life story. Thus, we should respect and honor whatever individuals choose for themselves. (p. 74)

H. Palliative Care

Wikipedia provides a comprehensive description of one of the sections in this book (Chapter 25 on the use of guided imagery and hypnosis for palliative care).

• Palliative care is a multidisciplinary approach to specialized medical and nursing care for people with life-limiting illnesses. It focuses on providing relief from the symptoms, pain, physical stress, and mental stress of a terminal diagnosis. The goal is to improve quality of life for both the person and their family.

- Palliative care is provided by a team of physicians, nurses, physiotherapists, occupational therapists, and other health professionals who work together with the primary care physician and referred specialists and other hospital or hospice staff to provide additional support. It is appropriate at any age and at any stage in a serious illness and can be provided as the main goal of care or along with curative treatment. Although it is an important part of end-of-life care, it is not limited to that stage. Palliative care can be provided across multiple settings including in hospitals, at home, as part of community palliative care programs, and in skilled nursing facilities. Interdisciplinary palliative care teams work with people and their families to clarify goals of care and provide symptom management, psycho-social, and spiritual support.

It is probably the case now that most hospitals have palliative care specialists on their staff. As indicated above, this is generally team work involving medical personnel with various specialties. Pain control is an obvious part of palliative care. At one time palliative care was *not* a part of hospice programs, but that has changed.

I. Death With Dignity Acts: Legal Programs in the United States

There are now several states in the U.S. that have legal death and dying programs administered by medical doctors. They are: Oregon, Washington, California, Colorado, Vermont, Montana, Washington DC, New Jersey, Maine, and Hawaii (many other states are considering this). A person who wishes to participate in such a program must be a legal resident of that state. Since the Oregon program is the oldest one in the U.S., I describe that program in some detail. Here is the link to their health department's annual report (latest one is 2020): www.oregon.gov/oha/ph/providerpartnerresources/evaluationresearch/deathwithdignityact. The Oregon program was the model, and all of the others in the U.S. are quite similar. (Non U.S. programs are quite different and are described separately in the next section.)

Oregon's Death with Dignity Act (DWDA) allows terminally ill adult Oregonians to obtain and use prescriptions from their physicians for self-administered, lethal doses of medications. The Oregon Public Health Division is required by the DWDA to collect compliance information and to issue an annual report. From its inception in 1998 to 2016 the annual number of deaths went from 16 to 133, and the annual number of prescription recipients from 24 to 204.

It is necessary to know how thoroughly the applicant is vetted before a prescription can be written. The person must be able to self-administer the drugs(s). The person also has to pay for the drugs personally, or in part or whole by their health insurance. Please note that the cost of these prescriptions is now considerable and may be between $3000 and $5000 U.S.

J. Death With Dignity Acts: Legal Programs in Other Countries

As of June 2019 human euthanasia is legal in The Netherlands, Belgium, Colombia, Luxembourg, and Canada. (FYI—The program in Canada is only for Canadian citizens, and operates primarily along the guidelines cited above for the Oregon one.) Only Switzerland will accept applicants who are not Swiss citizens. There are several such programs in Switzerland, and what follows are brief descriptions of them with contact information.

1 *Dignitas*—The costs of obtaining the assistance of Dignitas are of the order of $10,000 U.S., and do not include travel expenses. This cost may appear to be steep, but when all of the Dignitas services are considered it appears to be reasonable. The person must be capable of taking the medications, which are generally an oral dose of an anti-emetic drug, followed about 30 minutes later by a lethal overdose of 15 grams of powdered phenobarbital dissolved in a glass of water (www.dignitas.ch).
2 *Eternal Spirit Foundation*—The guiding principles of this foundation based in Basel, Switzerland are, "Eternal SPIRIT is committed to promote the legalization of assisted voluntary death in all countries. Eternal SPIRIT will analyze the applications for assisted voluntary death, which are made towards Eternal SPIRIT by members of lifecircle, and it will realize them when they are approved." *Application can only be made by members*. Their website is: www.lifecircle.ch. Please notice again, that the person must take the lethal medication themselves; if it is intravenously, they open the line (www.eternalspirit.ch).

B.4 Self-Deliverance

Self-deliverance (suicide) methods, or what I call Dying With Dignity, Choice, Control, Comfort, and Companionship, has been supported by the Hemlock society, Final Exit Network, and ERGO via the ad hoc NuTech committee for over 30 years. This committee meets sporadically and has done extensive research on methods that are quick, comfortable, and painless. Remember that suicide is not illegal, but assisting someone to do so is. Views on suicide have been influenced by broad existential themes such as religion, honor, and the meaning of life. The Abrahamic religions (Christian, Jewish, Islamic) traditionally consider suicide to be an offense towards God and the sanctity of life.

There are several books with information about self-deliverance methods:

1   Derek Humphry's *Final Exit* (2002)—This is the original book on the subject and contains practical information on many methods, and is in many editions.
2   Richard N. Cote's *In Search Of Gentle Death* (2012)—This is a journalist's history of the dying with dignity movement, and contains information on the history of the development of self-deliverance methods. There is much information on the NuTech Group.
3   Boudewijn Chabot's *A Way to Die* (2014)—The subtitle of this book is, "Methods for a Self-Chosen and Humane Death." Chabot is a medical doctor in The Netherlands. His book has a chapter on lethal drugs and another one on the helium method.
4   Chris Docker's *Five Last Acts—The Exit Path* (2013, 3rd Ed.)—The subtitle of this book is, "The arts and science of rational suicide in the face of unbearable, unrelievable suffering." This well-researched book is 752 pages long, of which the first 388 pages describe methods, and the remainder of the book are reference appendixes. Section 1, which is entitled "Last Acts," has five chapters: (1) Helium; (2) Compression (with a sub-section on drugs for self-deliverance); (3) Plastic bags with non-lethal drugs; (4) Lethal drug overdose; and (5) Fasting & other "fringe methods." (Docker is a leader of the Scottish EXIT group.)

I will provide some brief information in what follows on methods of self-deliverance. This will be about methods that are thoroughly described in the books cited above. In addition, the literature on the web also provides detailed information. This section is *strictly informative*, and in no way urges anyone to use any of the methods described as that is an individual choice. Some useful definitions are: *Suicide* is the act of taking one's own life; *Attempted suicide* is self-injury with the desire to end one's life that does not results in death; *Assisted suicide* is when one individual helps another bring about their own death directly or indirectly by persuading, urging, or coercing someone into committing suicide, or provides the means to an end and is illegal; and *Euthanasia* is where one person takes a more active role in bringing about a person's death.

A. Suicide Data for the United States

Since self-deliverance is actually suicide, it is important to understand its incidence and scope. Wikipedia's article on suicide in the U.S. is the source for the following information.

> Suicide is a major national social issue in the United States. In 2016, there were 44,965 recorded suicides, up from 42,773 in 2014, according to the CDC's National Center for Health Statistics. On average, adjusted for age, the annual U.S. suicide rate increased 24% between 1999 and 2014, from 10.5

to 13.0 suicides per 100,000 people, the highest rate recorded in 28 years. Due to the stigma surrounding suicide, it is suspected that it generally is under-reported.

In 2015, suicide was the seventh leading cause of death for males and the 14th leading cause of death for females. Additionally, it was the second leading cause of death for young people aged 15 to 24 and the third leading cause of death for those between the ages of 10 and 14. From 1999 to 2010, the suicide rate among Americans aged 35 to 64 increased nearly 30 per cent. The largest increases were among men in their fifties, with rates rising nearly 50 per cent, and for women aged 60 to 64, with rates rising 60 per cent. In 2008, it was observed that U.S. suicide rates, particularly among middle-aged white women, had increased, although the causes were unclear.

The U.S. ranks 48th in suicides/100,000 people at 12.6, with Sri Lanka the highest at 34.6. A good source for information and statistics is provided by the American Foundation for Suicide Prevention (https://afsp.org/about-suicide/suicide statistics). About 90% of people who commit suicide have a mental illness at the time of their death. Depression is the top risk factor, but there are various other mental health disorders that can contribute to suicide, including bipolar disorder and schizophrenia. In terms of method used, men are about twice as likely to use firearms as women, women are about three times as likely as men to use poison, and they both use suffocation and other methods at about the same rate.

B. Inert Gases: Helium and Nitrogen

The method involves feeding either pure helium or nitrogen gas into a small plastic bag (like a roasting bag) which is large enough to fit over the head comfortably. Once the bag is full, the person exhales fully and then pulls the bag over their head. The bag is kept in place with an elastic band (not tight). Enough of the gas then flows into the bag to ensure that the brain is starved of oxygen. Breathing then continues normally for both helium and nitrogen feel like air to breathe and do not cause any gasping for breath. Breathing will cease within minutes (it can be as quickly as 20 seconds). Complete death occurs shortly after the breathing ceases. Generally, the person becomes unconscious after one or two minutes, and dies after about three to five minutes. So, breathing in one of these non-reactive gases has no side effects, and rapidly induces a comfortable death.

C. Medications

The prescription medications used for assisted dying programs in the U.S. can only be obtained in those states after the vetting procedures described above. That is, *your medical doctor cannot prescribe them for your use.*

D. Voluntary Stopping Eating and Drinking (VSED)

This involves a decision to stop all eating and drinking, generally at the end of a terminal medical decline. It can be somewhat painful in the early stages unless the discomforts are alleviated with proper mouth care, thirst-reduction aids, pain relief for the underlying disease, or deep sedation. It generally takes 7 to 14 days before death occurs. This is for mentally competent patients who are terminally ill. *Palliative care and support is essential.* Generally, a hospice program will not accept a patient who declares that this is what they wish to do. However, once the person has started on this program and their life prognosis is certainly less than six months, then it is likely that their medical doctor can certify that they are eligible for hospice care. As noted in the emphasized words above, the kind of palliative care that is available in a hospice program would then become available.

E. Compression Method

This method (which is little known outside of Scotland) is discussed in great detail in Chapter 2 (pp. 179–243) in Docker's book (2013). It is something that an individual can do without assistance.

And, again, the mention of all the methods of self-deliverance mentioned in this book is simply informational.

B.5 Pain Control and Ideomotor Signaling

There are pain specialists available for end-of-life people who are suffering from cancer and other painful diseases. Hospice programs are excellent at pain control. One thing I learned from an expert (Joseph Barber) who uses hypnosis for pain control is to use *two* scales to assess how much a person is suffering. The first scale goes 0 to 10 where 0 is no pain at all and 10 is the most extreme pain the person has suffered or can imagine. The second scale is a *bother* one also goes from 0 to 10 where 0 is that the pain does not bother them at all, and 10 is that the pain is intolerably bothersome. So, a person may feel pain at a 7 level, but it only bothers them at a 3 level. Or, the pain may be at a level of 4, but it bothers them at an 8 level. It is also useful to indicate to the person that it is okay to use numbers like 3.7 and 8.5.

We generally have a good sense of our physical and mental condition. We can use ideomotor signaling (Rossi & Cheek, 1998; Cheek, 1994; Ewin & Eimer, 2006) to "ask" our bodies just what is going on at any given time. I do this and have taught others how to do this. An ideomotor signal is one that is autonomic and unconscious.

For this I designate the index finger on my right hand to be the "yes" finger, the middle finger to be the "no" finger, and my right thumb to be the "I am not ready to answer now" finger. Then, when I am relaxed with my eyes closed I just ask my body if a particular pain, for example, is something for me to worry about, and even perhaps call my doctor about. This is particularly important for someone who is in remission or undergoing treatment(s). At those times when a new (or old) pain occurs it may be a cause for worry. "Asking" your fingers to answer questions about how your body is doing can be quite helpful. Of course, when in doubt it is better to check with your doctor.

B.6 Dying and Living Well

It is said from time to time when you want to get back at someone who has done you harm in some way that the "best revenge" is to live a "good life." Living well should always be your goal. Revenge is living in the past and wasting your future. Just enjoy life and keep that person who wronged you out of it. I'm not saying forgive them or assist them in any way but just putting them and the event into its place will server you better. You will never teach them a lesson, and you will just be inflating their ego by giving them any attention. I know of too many people who have held grudges against a relative or friend for endless years. And, this is usually about something that happened a long time ago and that in perspective was probably not that important. Yet, we hold onto those insults or "dissings" (slang word for disrespect). So, either confront the person and attempt a reconciliation, or simply be a bit sad that they haven't changed. In my long life I have walked away feeling a bit sad from a number of relationships. There is a time to move on and live well.

The Bucket List is a movie that had an appropriate release on December 25, 2007. In it billionaire Edward Cole (Jack Nicholson) and car mechanic Carter Chambers (Morgan Freeman) are complete strangers, until fate lands them in the same hospital room. The men find they have two things in common: a need to come to terms with who they are and what they have done with their lives, and a desire to complete a list of things they want to see and do before they die. Against their doctor's advice, the men leave the hospital and set out on the adventure of a lifetime. A "bucket list" is a number of things you want to do before you die. "Kicking the bucket" is an idiom for dying. There are many theories as to where this idiom comes from, but the OED (Oxford English Dictionary) discusses the following: A person standing on a pail or bucket with their head in a slip noose would kick the bucket so as to commit suicide. Another explanation is from a Catholic custom that after death, when a body had been laid out ... the holy-water bucket was brought from the church and put at the feet of the corpse. When friends came to pray ... they would sprinkle the body with holy water and might accidentally "kick the bucket." At any rate, I hope you all have your own bucket lists and manage to arrange somehow to experience as many things on it of which you are capable.

Lawrence LeShan, a psychologist who worked with many "terminal" patients, found that when they took time towards the end of their lives to "sing their own song" that this activity brought meaning to their lives and that time. Joseph Campbell described this as finding and following your own "bliss." Viktor Frankl (1959, 1962, 1984) wrote about man's search for "meaning." These quests involve identifying your hopes, dreams, and unfulfilled desires. These all come under the title of "living well." That is, before that bucket shows up, fulfill some of those dreams.

I end this section with my desiderata for end-of-life:

Dying With Dignity, Choice, Control, Comfort, and Companions.

We do have choice, and there are places in this world where you can get assistance and/or guidance to die the way you want.

B.7 Some Closing Comments and References

LeShan (1990) has compiled a list of 33 significant questions for people in their dying time to consider. These questions are in Appendix C.

In a similar useful and practical manner you will find in Appendix D Bernie Siegel's (1986, pp. 127–128) *Patient's Bill of Rights*, which is written as an open letter to your physician(s).

This chapter has covered quite a few topics on end-of-life issues. For those of us getting closer to that time of life, or have a life-challenging disease, I trust that you will have found enough significant material and ideas and references to help you through this part of your life. As I indicated in the Preface to this book, my volunteer work for many years has been in this area. In the past two years, six of my closest friends—people I have known for 40 to 70 years—have died. Recently, three men and two women I have known as friends in my small town have also died. So, this is personal to me, and is also universal.

Addendum I: Writing

My mother died of lung cancer many years ago, and it took me a long time to come to grips with her death and that loss. At that time, the word cancer was always *whispered* (just in case an evil spirit heard it and would give it to you). Everyone in my family (my father and my four siblings) knew that she had cancer. I had read Elisabeth Kübler-Ross (1969, 1975) on death and dying around then and decided that, despite my family's misgivings, I would have a frank discussion with my mother on the evening before she had her lung surgery. My father was in a lounge down the hall, and she and I could talk privately. I told her I knew that she had cancer, and wondered if we could talk about it. I was surprised to hear her say, "Of course I know I have cancer—I know my body." We had an amazingly intimate chat in which she told me that she had dreams of two places she would like to visit before she died. The first was that she wanted to go to Florida since she had heard so much about it. For the second, I note my father was the salesman for the small pajama and nightgown company in which he was a partner. As such, he traveled to Boston regularly. My mother wanted to see Boston! That was the last time I saw her alive. She survived the surgery, but died a few months later (August 16, 1976). So how did I, in my forties then, handle this?

There was an interesting man who lived in our tenement in the Bronx. His name was Mr. Meyers, and it turned out that his favorite philosopher was Spinoza. He read Spinoza's writings all of the time. I did not know how to come to grips with my mother's death for about two years, when I had an idea. By that time I had already written a few plays.[2] I started writing a play that featured a Mr. Meyers who was an old Jewish man dying of cancer in a hospital. In the course of the play Mr. Meyers, who is a kind of comic philosopher, teaches everyone around him both how to live and how to die. He also helped me cope with my mother's death. I had a friend at the time named Al Radin who actually grew up in the area of the Bronx where I did. He still had a pronounced "Noo Yawk" accent. So, scene by scene, I imagined Mr. Meyers talking to me with Al's accent so I could write with correct New York accents and rhythms. (The play is entitled *The Local Train*.)

What is the relevance of the previous story? When I lead sessions using the Remen healing circle with its small smooth flat stones, I first model what each volunteer (or person in the circle) would say. I tell the audience what helped me get over a particularly difficult time in my life was writing, and that was what I put in the stone for that group for a particular member. So, writing is the special way I use for coping with and living with troubling and difficult times in my life. This chapter has to do with end-of-life issues, and I am going to share with you here a number of my three-line poems. I start with poems dedicated to a number of members of the Charlie Brown support group, all of whom died from cancer.

Art Teacher
her head bald from chemo
is painted with bright blue flowers
and glows from within

Anna
Anna is dying
straggly hair, yellow-tinged face
eyes still bright, alive
I held her warm hand

spasmodic with the drugs
sending love

Lu
Lu is dying, too
talking too much as usual
soaking in the sunset

Bill
Bill's pain is my pain
errant cells multiplying
his bravery mine

Carolyn
caught by cancer
she never gives up hope
Carolyn smoking

Janet
fighting the cancer
her smile illuminates the room
Janet just being

quiet dignity
through the nausea and the pain
Janet's inner peace

The following two series were about friends of mine who contacted me early in their diagnosis of having cancer. I met with them (and their husbands) frequently over periods of three years. Both sets were written while at their bedsides just short times before they died.

Mary
can I breathe with you
while you lie there comatose
spirit to spirit

through her haze she said
I am only twenty per cent here
Mary dying ...

at the end of life
rest home with stuffed animals
tremors and sleep

breathing softly
she sleeps in a peaceful coma
still full of dreams

mostly sleeping now
Mary of the peace marches
continues to witness

with her strong hands
she molds another earthen image
for Potters for Peace[3]

forever smiling
Mary radiates love
friend to friend to friend

Dotti
Dotti, still a mother
consoles her crying husband
from her cancer bed

her lingering smile
shone through the waves of pain
Dotti's courage

Gary the poet
records his and Dotti's struggle
in vivid images

Hospice of Dayton
trees and geese and ducks
the greening of dying

When he died in November 2017, George was my oldest living friend. We met in our freshman year in high school and kept contact over the years. I wrote the following six poems, which were read at his celebration of life memorial service. His family wanted him to be a dentist, but the theater called him. He and his wife, Gilda, both got immersed in theater, and George had a super career as a director, actor, and professor of theater.

George
George is gone
how convey the sadness, the emptiness
I write ...

the director has left us
his raspy voice talking

the words filling my soul

that forceful energy
positive, loving, teaching
engraved deep within me

always opinionated
discoursing profoundly
the director has left us

we were students together
learners and hikers and dreamers
and now ...

my brother George
is no more
memories sustain me

When my father died peacefully at 94 I saw him that afternoon. Afterwards I simply wrote:

the old man is gone
his hopes and dreams
quietly passing in the night

And, most recently, my oldest brother, Ralph, died peacefully on March 23, 2019 well into his hundredth year. When I heard in late afternoon that he had opted for risky surgery so he could walk again rather than never walk again, these words came to me in the middle of that night:

I do mundane things
while brother Ralph may be dying
I am, am I?

He died the next day from a blood clot (after having survived the surgery). Then, I wrote:

brother Ralph is gone
his smile and laughter lingering
the silence of sorrow

Addendum 2: Henning Mankell's Wisdom

Henning George Mankell was a Swedish crime writer, children's author, and dramatist, best known for a series of detective novels starring his most noted creation, Inspector Kurt Wallander. He also wrote a number of plays and screenplays for television. He was a left-wing social critic and activist. He was born in 1948, and died in 2015. The following are some quotes from his book *Quicksand* (Mankell, 2017). He wrote this book when he received a diagnosis of cancer, and in his last year of life. I found them to be quite meaningful.

Being stricken by cancer is an extreme catastrophe. ... The only thing I am quite clear about is being convinced that time has stood still. As if in a concentrated and condensed universe, everything has become a point in which there was no past or future: nothing but now. I was a human being clinging fast to the edge of a patch of death-bringing quicksand.

(pp. 16–17)

Once you are dead, you are dead. You can no longer influence earthly things. Being alive is being able to say yes or no. Being dead is to be surrounded by silence.

(p. 25)

While you remain in somebody's memory, you still have your identity. But eventually that fades away as well. ... It is man's fate to be forgotten.

(pp. 83–84)

Fear is natural and based on the simple truth that what distinguishes humans from other species is that we know we are going to die. The cats I have owned during my life have never been aware of their own death.

(p. 94)

Facing up to cancer is a battle conducted on many fronts. The important thing is not to waste too much strength fighting against one's own illusions. I need all my strength in order to increase my powers of resistance in confronting the enemy that has invaded me. Not tilting at windmills that have taken on the form of shadows.

(p. 119)

Life is short. But death is very very long. "How long is eternity?" asks the child. Who can answer that question?

(p. 144)

My deepest fear is something quite different. Silly, childish. I'm afraid of being dead for such a long time. It is a pointless fear, almost embarrassing. In death there is no time, no space, no anything. My role in the long-dance of

death will be over. I shall have fallen off the staircase of life on the final step.
... But perhaps that is the most confidence-inspiring aspect of death?

(p. 193)

Living with cancer means living with no guarantees.

(p. 268)

At that time it never occurred to me that love is a blessing – perhaps the greatest blessing a human being can be gifted with. It was only later that thought came into my mind.

(p. 278)

(Epilogue) All these unknown people exist alongside me. For a short time they have been part of my life. I share it with all of them. Our real family is endless, even if we don't know who some of them were when we met them for an extremely brief moment.

(p. 303)

To: All of you who have gone before and shared some of your

lives with me, and who have enriched me

and populated my memory banks

with love and joy and laughter—Thank You

Addendum 3: Books that Have Influenced My Volunteer Work

- LeShan, L. (1977). *You can fight for your life. Emotional factors in the treatment of cancer.* This older book describes LeShan's pioneering work in spending time with people who have cancer. When LeShan asked doctors if he could work with cancer patients, they said "yes," but only with *terminal* ones! That is, they figured he could not do any harm to them.
- LeShan, L. (1990). *Cancer as a turning point. A handbook for people with cancer, their families, and health professionals.* This is a wonderful book, even though it is a bit dated.
- Bolletino, R. C. (2009). *How to talk with family caregivers about cancer.* This is an excellent book, and is based on her many years of being mentored by LeShan. There is much useful practical advice for caregivers.
- Buckman, R. (1992). *How to break bad news. A guide for health care professionals.* Buckman was a pioneer in the use of language with people who have life-challenging diseases. This is a must-read book in this area.

- Remen, R. N. (1996). *Kitchen table wisdom. Stories that heal.* Remen is the medical director of Commonweal, a residential place for people who have cancer and other serious ailments. Her stories are healing.
- Hammerschlag, C. A. & Silverman, H. D. (1997). *Healing ceremonies. Creating personal rituals for spiritual, emotional, physical and mental health.* This book tells the stories of people who have confronted health problems and life events with powerful personal ceremonies. It is a primer on healing ceremonies.

Notes

1 I am ignoring here all of those people who believe in reincarnation or whose religious beliefs guarantee (most of!) them a life after death in some kind of heaven.
2 Incidentally, the first play I wrote was entitled *Marathon*, and was based on a marathon Gestalt Therapy group session with three therapists and ten clients, and which lasted 24 hours! I have written a bunch of plays, some psychotherapy books, many technical papers, and a whole bunch of three-line poems.
3 Mary founded the organization Potters for Peace.

Appendix C: Questions for People in Their Dying Time

Lawrence LeShan has compiled a list of 33 significant questions for people in their dying time to consider (1990, pp. 161–165). These are good questions to ponder at any time of your life. You may find these questions to be useful in organizing your thinking and considering your life. You may wish to share your responses with a compassionate friend or relative, or write your responses in your journal.

1 As you look at your whole life from the viewpoint of where you are now, what was it all about? Was it a good life? Was it a lonely life? Was it a frustrating life?

2 If your whole life had been designed in advance so that you would learn something from it, what would be the lesson you were supposed to have learned? Did you really learn it? What else would you have needed in order to have learned it?

3 What was the best thing that ever happened to you? What was the worst? (These are separate questions and, as a general rule, seem to be the most helpful when asked in this order.)

4 What was the best thing you ever did? What was the worst?

5 What was the best period of your life? What was the worst?

6 How would you finish these statements: "Out of my childhood I love to remember …" "Out of my childhood I hate to remember …"?

7 Do you believe it is true that "It is better to have loved and lost than never to have loved at all?" What led you to this conclusion?

8 If you were asked by a child you love to tell him or her the one most important thing that you have learned in life, what would you reply?

9 There is an old Greek legend about the three Fates who govern all lives: Clotho, who weaves the thread of a person's life; Lachesis, who colors it; and Atropos, who cuts it and the person dies. How did Lachesis color *your* life? Did Atropos cut it off too soon? Too soon for what? Can you still do what you have unfinished so far?

10 In each symphony (ballad, folk song, popular song) there is a central theme. It has many variations, these appear in the different sections

(verses), but underlying them all is the theme. What has been the theme of your life?

11 If you could change *one decision* of your life, what would it be? Why did you make it the way you did? What does this tell you about how you saw yourself and the world at that time? Can you forgive yourself for making that decision the way you did? For feeling the way you did? If not, why?

12 For the things you did, what do you now need to do in order to be able to forgive yourself?

13 For the things that others did to you, what do you need to do in order to forgive them? For the things that happened to you, what do you need in order to forgive yourself?

14 If you were to overhear your friends talking about you at your funeral, what would you most like to hear them say about you? Like least to hear?

15 As you look back on your life, what were the moments when you were most yourself? What helped you to do this? What were the moments you were least yourself? Why do you think this was so?

16 What was the best time of your life? Tell me about it? What was the worst time of your life? Tell me about it.

17 How were you the same all your life, as a child, a youth, an adult, now? How were you different at those different times of your life?

18 What do you need to finish your life, to complete it? Can you do it from this hospital room?

19 During this time, what is the longest time of the day for you? What do you mostly feel and think during this time?

20 In an ancient manuscript *The Book of Splendor* is the statement: "God's purpose is not to add years to your life, but to add life to your years." What do you think of this?

21 What is the thing in yourself that you have been most afraid to experience consciously? To think and feel about? Does it now seem as necessary to hide it from yourself as it did in the past?

22 What is it about you that you have most hidden from others? Does it seem as necessary to keep it hidden as it did in the past?

23 All our lives we try to change people to what we think they should be. At this time of life we can often see that love is accepting people as they are and letting them be while hoping and wishing for more for them. Can you do this with those you love? What in you keeps you from this?

24 The time of dying is the last learning time we have on Earth. What lesson is there for you to learn in your dying? What in you keeps you from being able to learn it?

25 What is the major role you have played in recent years? What masks have you worn most often in the presence of others? Are they roles you wish to play during these last times?

26 All our lives we try to *accomplish* something, to *do* something. What is it that you were trying to do in recent years? Is it still so important to you? How can you finish the attempt so that it ends with the most harmony and honesty?

27 Have you been mostly walking one road in recent years? Is there another road that you now need to walk in order to make your life journey more complete?

28 Is there someone you protected in recent years at a high cost in energy and time? Are you still trying to protect him or her? (Or be something for him or her?) Is it the best thing for this person for you to continue protecting him or her? For you?

29 What do you need to *finish* your life? Can you do it from this bed? How or why not? It is in *you* that we need to finish things and it is inside you that you can.

30 What is it that has happened to you that you have never been able to forgive God (or the Fates) for?

31 For what do you most need the forgiveness of God?

32 There is the story of one of the great Hasidic Rabbis named Zusya. His congregation asked him to do something, a particular political action. He refused. They said, "If Moses were our Rabbi, he would do it." Zusya answered, "When I die and rise and stand before the throne, God will not ask me why I was not Moses. He will ask me why I was not Zusya." Does this story in any way relate to you and your life? How?

33 What has been the best season of the year for you? Why?

Appendix D: Patient's Bill of Rights

Bernie Siegel (1986, pp. 127–128) gives the following as a patient's bill of rights. It is written as an open letter to physicians.

Dear Doctor:

Please don't conceal the diagnosis. We both know I came to you to learn if I have cancer or some other serious disease. If I know what I have, I know what I am fighting, and there is less to fear. If you hide the name and the facts, you deprive me of the chance to help myself. When you are questioning whether I should be told, I already know. You may feel better if you don't tell me, but your deception hurts.

Do not tell me how long I have to live! I alone can decide how long I will live. It is my desires, my goals, my values, my strengths, and my will to live that will make the decision.

Teach me and my family about how and why my illness happened to me. Help me and my family to live *now*. Tell me about nutrition and my body's needs. Tell me how to handle the knowledge and how my mind and body can work together. Healing comes from within, but I want to combine my strength with yours. If you and I are a team, I will live a longer and better life.

Doctor, don't let your negative beliefs, your fears, and your prejudices affect my health. Don't stand in the way of my getting well and exceeding your expectations. Give me the chance to be the exception to your statistics.

Teach me about your beliefs and therapies and help me to incorporate them into mine. However, remember that my beliefs are the most important. What I don't believe in won't help me.

You must learn what my disease means to me—death, pain, or fear of the unknown. If my belief system accepts alternative therapy and not recognized therapy, do not desert me. Please try to convert to my beliefs, and be patient and await my conversion. It may come at a time when I am desperately ill and in great need of your therapy.

Doctor, teach me and my family to live with my problem when I am not with you. Take time for our questions and give us your attention when we need it. It is important that I feel free to talk with you and question you. I will live a longer and more meaningful life if you and I can develop a significant relationship. I need you in my life to achieve my new goals.

References

Achterberg, J. (1985). *Imagery in healing: shamanism and modern medicine.* Boston: New Science Library.

Achterberg, J., Dossey, B., & Kolkmeier, L. (1994). *Rituals of healing: using imagery for health and wellness.* New York: Bantam Books.

Andreas, C., & Andreas, S. (1989). *Heart of the mind. Engaging your inner power to change with neuro-linguistic programming.* Moab, UT: Real People Press.

Andreas, S. (2012). *Transforming negative self-talk. Practical, effective exercises.* New York: W. W. Norton & Company.

Andreas, S. (2014a). *More transforming negative self-talk. Practical, effective exercises.* New York: W. W. Norton & Company.

Andreas, S. (2014b). SST with NLP: Rapid transformations using content-free instructions. In Hoyt, M. F., and Talmon, M. (Eds.). *Capturing the moment. Single session therapy and walk-in services.* (pp. 277–298). Carmarthen, UK: Crown House Publishing Ltd.

Anonymous (1992). *Alternative medicine: expanding medical horizons. A report to the National Institutes of Health on alternative medical systems and practices in the United States.* [Prepared under the auspices of the Workshop on alternative Medicine, Chantilly, Virginia, September 14–16, 1992. Order from: Superintendent of Documents, 017-040-00537-7. U.S. Government Printing Office.]

Bandler, R., & Grinder, J. (1975). *The structure of magic I. A book about language and therapy.* Palo Alto, CA: Science and Behavior Books.

Bank, W. O. (1985). Hypnotic suggestion for the control of bleeding in the angiography suite. In S. R. Lankton (Ed.), *Ericksonian Monographs No. 1. Elements and Dimensions of an Ericksonian Approach.* (pp. 76–88). New York: Brunner/Mazel.

Barber, J. & Adrian, C. (1982). (Eds.). *Psychological approaches to the management of pain.* New York: Brunner/Mazel.

Barber, J. (1996). (Ed.). *Hypnosis and suggestion in the treatment of pain. A clinical guide.* New York: W.W. Norton & Company.

Battino, R. & South, T. L. (1st Ed. 1997, 2nd Ed. 2005). *Ericksonian approaches. A comprehensive manual.* Carmarthen, UK: Crown House Publishing Ltd.

Battino, R. (2000). *Guided imagery and other approaches to healing.* Carmarthen, UK: Crown House Publishing Ltd.

Battino, R. (2001). *Coping. A practical guide for people with life-challenging diseases and their caregivers.* Carmarthen, UK: Crown House Publishing Ltd.

Battino, R. (2002). *Meaning: A Play Based on the Life of Viktor E. Frankl.* Williston, CT: Crown House Publishing.

Battino, R. (2002). *Metaphoria. Metaphor and guided metaphor for psychotherapy and healing.* Carmarthen, UK: Crown House Publishing Ltd.

Battino, R. (2006). *Expectation. The very brief therapy book.* Carmarthen, UK: Crown House Publishing Ltd.

Battino, R. (2007). *Guided imagery: Psychotherapy and healing through the mind-body connection.* Bethel, CT: Crown House Publishing.

Battino, R. (2007). *That's right, is it not? A play about the life of Milton H. Erickson, M.D.* Phoenix, AZ: Milton H. Erickson Foundation Press.

Battino, R. (2010). *Healing language. A guide for physicians, dentists, nurses, psychologists, social workers, and counselors.* (Available from Lulu.com & Amazon.com)

Battino, R. (2014). Expectation: The essence of very brief therapy. In M. F. Hoyt & M. Talmon (Eds.), *Capturing the Moment: Single-Session Therapy and Walk-In Services* (pp. 393–406). Bethel, CT: Crown House Publishing.

Battino, R. (2015). *When all else fails. Some new and some old tools for doing brief therapy.* Carmarthen, UK: Crown House Publishing Ltd.

Benedetti, F., Lanotte, M., Lopiano, L., & Colloca, L. (2007). (Review) When words are painful: unraveling the mechanisms of the nocebo effect. *Neuroscience, 147,* 260–271.

Berne, E. (1964). *Games people play–the basic handbook of transactional analysis.* New York: Ballantine Books.

Bolletino, R. C. (2009). *How to talk with family caregivers about cancer.* New York: W. W. Norton & Company.

Buckman, R. (1992). *How to break bad news. A guide for health care professionals.* Baltimore: The Johns Hopkins University Press.

Buckman, R. (1988). *I don't know what to say-how to hep & support someone who is dying.* Toronto: Key Porter.

Byock, I. (2004). *The four things that matter most in life. A book about living.* New York: Free Press.

Chabot, B. (2014). *A way to die. Methods for a self-chosen and humane death.* Amsterdam, Netherlands: Foundation Dignified Dying.

Cheek, D. B. (1959). Unconscious perception of meaningful sounds during surgical anesthesia as revealed under hypnosis. *American Journal of Clinical Hypnosis, 1,* 101–113.

Cheek, D. B. (1960a). Use of preoperative hypnosis to protect patients from careless conversation. *American Journal of Clinical Hypnosis, 3*(2), 101–102.

Cheek, D. B. (1960b). What does the surgically anesthetized patient hear? *Rocky Mountain Medical Journal, 57,* January, 49–53.

Cheek, D. B. (1961). Unconscious reactions and surgical risk. *Western Journal of Surgery, Obstetrics, and Gynecology, 69,* 325–328.

Cheek, D. B. (1964). Further evidence of persistence of hearing under chem-anesthesia: detailed case report. *American Journal of Clinical Hypnosis, 7*(1), 55–59.

Cheek, D. B. (1965). Can surgical patients react to what they hear under anesthesia? *Journal American Association Nurse Anesthetists, 33,* 30–38.

Cheek, D. B. (1966). The meaning of continued hearing sense under general anesthesia, *American Journal of Clinical Hypnosis, 8,* 275–280.

Cheek, D. B. (1981). Awareness of meaningful sounds under general anesthesia: considerations and a review of the literature. In H. J. Wain, *Theoretical and Clinical Aspects of Hypnosis*: Miami: Symposia Specialists Inc.

Cheek, D.B. (1994). *Hypnosis: The application of ideomotor procedures.* Boston: Allyn & Bacon.

Clance, P. R. (1985). *The impostor phenomenon: overcoming the fear that haunts your success.* Harrisonburg, VA: Donnelley Printing Co.

Clawson, T. A., & Swade, R. H. (1975). The hypnotic control of blood flow and pain: the cure of warts and the potential for the use of hypnosis in the treatment of cancer. *American Journal of Clinical Hypnosis, 17*, 160–169.

Colloca, L. (2017). Nocebo effects can make you feel pain. *Science, 358*, 44.

Colloca, L., & Benedetti, F. (2005). Placebos and painkillers: is mind as real as matter? *Neuroscience, 6*, 545–552.

Colloca, L., & Benedetti, F. (2006). How prior experience shapes placebo analgesia. *Pain, 124*, 126–133.

Colloca, L., & Benedetti, F. (2007). Nocebo hyperalgesia: how anxiety is turned into pain. *Current Opinions in Anesthesiology, 20*, 435–439.

Cote, R. N. (2012). *In search of gentle death. The fight for your right to die with dignity*. Mt. Pleasant, South Carolina: Corinthian Books.

Cousins, N. (1979, 1981). *Anatomy of an illness*. New York: W. W. Norton & Co.

Czobor, P., & Skolnick, P. (2011). The secrets of a successful clinical trial: compliance, compliance, and compliance. *Molecular Interventions, 11*, 107–110.

Docker, C. (2013). (3rd Ed.) *Five last acts – the exit path*. (Published by Exit. 17 Hart Street, Edinburgh, EH1 3RN, Scotland, U.K.

Dubin, L. L., & Shapiro, S. S. (1974). Use of hypnosis to facilitate dental extraction and homeostasis in a classic hemophiliac with a high antibody titer to Factor VIII. *American Journal of Clinical Hypnosis, 17*, 79–83.

Erickson, M. H. & Rossi, E. L. (1989). *The February man. Evolving consciousness and identity in hypnotherapy*. New York: Brunner/Mazel.

Esdaille, J. (1846, 1902). *Mesmerism in India and its practical application in surgery and medicine*. London: Long, Brown, Green and Longmans. [1902 edition available from Amazon.com.]

Ewin, D. M. & Eimer, B. N. (2006). *Ideomotor signals for rapid hypnoanalysis. A how-to manual*. Springfield, IL: Charles C. Thomas Publisher.

Enck, P., Benedetti, F., & Schedlowski, M. (2008). New insights into the placebo and nocebo responses. *Neuron, 59*, 195–206.

Epston, D., & White, M. (1992). *Experience, contradiction, narrative & imagination. Selected papers of David Epston & Michael White (1989–1991)*. Dulwich Centre Publications (Hutt St. P.O. Box 7192, Adelaide, 5000, South Australia).

Farrelly, F., & Brandsma, J. (1974). *Provocative therapy*. Millbrae, CA: Celestial Arts, Shields Publishing Co., Inc.

Fink, H. H. & Battino, R. (2011). *Howie and Ruby. Conversations 2000–2007*. (Available from Lulu.com & Amazon.com)

Finniss, D. G., Kaptchuk, T. J., Miller, F., & Benedetti, F. (2010). Biological, clinical, and ethical advances of placebo effects. (Review). *Lancet, 375*, 686–695.

Frankl, V. E. (1959; 1962 Rev. Ed.; 1984 3rd Ed.) *Man's search for meaning*. New York: Simon and Schuster.

Freedman, J. & Combs, G. (1996). *Narrative therapy. The social construction of preferred realities*. New York: W. W. Norton & Co.

Gifford, K. D. (1998). The Mediterranean diet as a food guide: the problem of culture and history. *Nutrition Today, 33*, 233–243.

Grinder, J., & Bandler, R. (1976). *The structure of magic II*. Palo Alto, CA: Science and Behavior Books.

Hahn, R. A. (1997). *The nocebo phenomenon: scope and foundations*. In A. Harrington (Ed.), *The placebo effect. An interdisciplinary exploration*. (pp. 56–76) Cambridge, MA: Harvard University Press.

Hammerschlag, C. A. (1988). *The dancing healers.* New York: Harper-Collins.

Hammerschlag, C. A. (1993). *The theft of the spirit.* New York: Simon & Schuster.

Hammerschlag, C. A. & Silverman, H. D. (1997). *Healing ceremonies. Creating personal rituals for spiritual, emotional, physical and mental health.* New York: A Perigree Book (The Berkley Publishing Group).

Hill, R., & Rossi, E. L. (2017). *The practitioner's guide to mirroring hands. A client-responsive therapy that facilitates natural problem solving and mind-body healing.* Carmarthen, UK: Crown House Publishing Ltd.

Hillman, H. (2013). *The imposter syndrome. Becoming an authentic leader.* New Zealand: Random House.

Hoyt, M. F. (1995). *Brief therapies and managed care.* San Francisco: Jossey-Bass.

Hoyt, M. F. (2000). *Some stories are better than others. Doing what works in brief therapy and managed care.* Philadelphia: Brunner/Mazel.

Hoyt, M. F. (2004). *The present is a gift: mo' better stories from the world of brief therapy.* New York: iUniverse, Inc.

Hoyt, M. (2009). *Brief therapies. Principles & practices.* Phoenix, AZ: Zeig, Tucker & Theisen, Inc.

Hoyt, M. F., and Talmon, M. (2014). (Eds.). *Capturing the moment. Single session therapy and walk-in services.* Carmarthen, UK: Crown House Publishing Ltd.

Hoyt, M. F. (2017). *Brief therapy and beyond. Stories, language, love, hope, and time.* New York: Routledge.

Hoyt, M. F., Bobele, M., Slive, A., Young, J., & Talmon, M. (2018). (Eds.). *Single-Session Therapy by Walk-in or Appointment.* New York: Routledge.

Hoyt, M. F. & Bobele, M. (Eds.). (2019). *Creative therapy in challenging situations. Unusual interventions to help clients.* New York: Routledge.

Humphry, D. (1978, 2003). *Jean's Way,* Junction City, OR: Norris Lane Press.

Humphry, D. (1981). *Let me die before I wake: Hemlock's book of self-deliverance and assisted suicide for the dying.* Los Angeles: The Hemlock Society.

Humphry, D., & Wickett, A. (1986). *The right to die: understanding euthanasia.* New York: Harper & Row Publishers.

Humphry, D. (1991). *Euthanasia: help with a good death. Essays and briefings on the right to choose to die.* Eugene, OR: Hemlock Society.

Humphry, D. (1992). *Dying with dignity: understanding euthanasia.* Secaucus, NJ: Carol Publishing Group.

Humphry, D. (1992). *Rational suicide among the elderly.* New York: Guildford Press.

Humphry, D., & Clement, M. (1998, 2000). *Freedom to die: people, politics, and the right-to-die movement.* New York: St. Martin's Press.

Humphry, D. (2002). *Final exit. The practicalities of self-deliverance and assisted suicide for the dying.* (3rd Ed.) Eugene, OR: The Hemlock Society (P.O. Box 11830, Eugene, OR 97440). (also; New York: Random House - 2010.)

Humphry, D. (2004, 2005, 2006). *The good euthanasia guide. Where, what, and who in the choices in dying.* Junction City, OR: Norris Lane Press/ERGO.

Humphry, D. (2008). *Good life, good death: a memoir.* Junction City, OR: Norris Lane Press/ERGO.

Jin, J., Sklar, G. E., Sen Oh, V. M., & Li, S. C. (2008). Factors affecting therapeutic compliance: a review from the patient's perspective. *Therapeutic Clinical Risk Management, 4,* 269–286.

Kane, S., & Olness, K. (eds.), 2004, *The art of therapeutic communication: the collected works of Kay F. Thompson.* Carmarthen, UK: Crown House Publishing.

Kopp, S. B. (1972). *If you meet the Buddha on the road, kill him! The pilgrimage of psychotherapy patients*. Ben Lomond, CA: Science and Behavior Books, Inc.

Kübler-Ross, E. (1969). *On death and dying*. New York: Macmillan.

Kübler-Ross, E. (1975). *Death, the final stage of growth*. Englewood Cliffs, NJ: Prentice-Hall.

L'Abate, L., & Cox, J. (1992). *Programmed writing: A self-administered approach for interventions with individuals, couples, and families*. Pacific Grove, CA: Brooks/Cole.

L'Abate, L. (2004). (Ed.). *Using workbooks in mental health. Resources in prevention, psychotherapy, and rehabilitation for clinicians and researchers*. New York: The Haworth Press, Inc.

Laing, R. D. (1970). *Knots*. New York: Pantheon Books (Random House).

Lankton, S. R. & Lankton, C. H. (1986). *Enchantment and intervention in family therapy. Training in Ericksonian approaches*. New York: Brunner/Mazel.

Lee, B. C. (2019). *Finish strong. Putting your priorities first at life's end*. Littelton, CO: Compassion & Choices (see: FinishStronginfo@CompassionandChoices.org).

LeShan, L. (1977). *You can fight for your life. Emotional factors in the treatment of cancer*. New York: M. Evans and Company, Inc.

LeShan, L. (1990). *Cancer as a turning point. A handbook for people with cancer, their families, and health professionals*. New York: Plume (Penguin Group).

Levine, S. (1997). *A year to live. How to live your life as if it were the last*. New York: Bell Tower. (Crown Publishing Group.)

Lindner, R. (1955). *The fifty-minute hour. A collection of true psychoanalytic tales*. New York: Bantam Books.

Liu, W. H. D., Standen, P. J., & Aitkenhead, A. R. (1992). Therapeutic suggestions during general anesthesia in patients undergoing hysterectomy. *British Journal of Anesthesia*, 68, 277–281.

Mankell, H. (2017). *Quicksand: what it means to be a human being*. New York: Vintage Books.

Meichenbaum, D. & Turk, D. C. (1987). *Facilitating treatment adherence; a practitioner's guidebook*. New York: Plenum Press.

Miller, S. D., & Berg, I. K. (1995). *The miracle method. A radically new approach to problem drinking*. New York: W.W. Norton & Company.

Miller, F. G., & Colloca, L. (2009). The legitimacy of placebo treatments in clinical practice: evidence and ethics. *The American Journal of Bioethics*, 9, 39–47.

Milstein, L. B. (1994, 2004). *Giving comfort. What you can do when someone you know is ill*. New York: Penguin Books.

Naparstek, B. (1995). *Staying well with guided imagery*. New York: Warner Books Inc.

Naparstek, B., & Scaer, R. C. (2005). *Invisible heroes: survivors of trauma and how they heal*. New York: Bantam Dell.

Naparstek, B. (2009). *Your sixth sense: unlocking the power of your mind (plus)*. New York: HarperCollins Publishers.

Nardone, G., and Portelli, C. (2005). *Knowing through changing: the evolution of brief strategic therapy*. Carmarthen, UK: Crown House Publishing Ltd.

Norcross, J. C., & Wampold, B. E. (2011). Evidence-based therapy relationships: Research conclusions and clinical practices. *Psychotherapy*, 48, 98–102.

Ornish, D. (1991). *Dr. Dean Ornish's program for reversing heart disease*. New York: Ballantine Books.

Pearson, R. E. (1961). Response to suggestions given under general anesthesia. *American Journal of Clinical Hypnosis*, 4, 106–114.

Pennebaker, J. W. (1997). "Writing about emotional experiences as a therapeutic process." *Psychological Science*, 8, pp. 162–166.

Pennebaker, J. W., and Chung, C. K. (2007). "Expressive writing, emotional upheavals, and health." In H. Friedman and B. Silver (Eds.), *Handbook of Health Psychology*. pp. 263–284. New York: Oxford University Press.

Rainwater, J. (1979). *You're in charge! A guide to becoming your own therapist.* Los Angeles: Guild of Tutors.

Remen, R. N. (1996). *Kitchen table wisdom. Stories that heal.* New York: Riverhead Books.

Rossi, E. L. (2002). *The psychobiology of gene expression: neuroscience and neurogenesis in hypnosis and the healing arts.* New York: W. W. Norton.

Rossi, E. L., & Cheek, D. B. (1988). *Mind-body therapy. Ideodynamic healing in hypnosis.* New York: W. W. Norton & Co.

Schneider, S. H. (2005). *The patient from hell. How I worked with my doctors to get the best of modern medicine and HOW YOU CAN TOO.* Boston: Da Capo Lifelong Books (Hatchette Book Group).

Seligman, M. E. P. (2003). *Authentic happiness: using the new positive psychology to realize your potential for lasting fulfillment.* New York: The Free Press (Simon & Schuster, Inc.).

Shapiro, A.S. (2009). *Healing into possibility. The transformational lessons of a stroke.* Novato, CA: New World Library.

Shapiro, A. K., & Shapiro, E. (1997). *The powerful placebo. From ancient to modern times.* Baltimore: The Johns Hopkins University Press.

Siegel, B. S. (1986). *Love, medicine & miracles. Lessons learned about self-healing from a surgeon's experience with exceptional patients.* New York: HarperPerennial (HarperCollins Publishers).

Siegel, B.S. (1989). *Peace, love & healing. Bodymind communication & the path to self-healing: an exploration.* New York: Harper & Row.

Siegel, B.S. (1993). *How to live between office visits. A guide to life, love and health.* New York: HarperCollins.

Siegel, B.S. (2013). *The art of healing. Uncovering your inner wisdom and potential for self-healing.* Novato, CA: New World Library.

Silvester, T. (2003). *Wordweaving. The science of suggestion. A comprehensive guide to creating hypnotic language.* Berkekey House: Cippenham, Slough, Berks, England. (First published by The Quest Institute.)

Silvester, T. (2006). *Wordweaving. Vol. II. The question is the answer. Focusing on solutions with cognitive therapy.* England, Old Ness Farm, Ness Road, Burwell, Cambs, CB5 0DB. (First published by The Quest Institute.)

Silvester, T. (2010). *Cognitive hypnotherapy: "What's that about and how can I use it?"* Leicester, UK: Matador. (www.troubador.co.uk/matador)

Simonton, O. C., Simonton, S. M., & Creighton, J. (1980). *Getting well again.* New York: Bantam Books.

Simonton, S. M. (1984). *The healing family. The Simonton approach for families facing illness.* New York: Bantam Books.

Talmon, M. (1990). *Single session therapy. Maximizing the effect of the first (and often only) therapeutic encounter.* San Francisco: Jossey-Bass Publishers.

Thomas, K. B. (1987). General practice consultations: is there any point in being positive? *British Medical Journal, 294*, 1200–1202.

Thompson, K. F. (1976). A clinical view of the effectiveness of hypnosis in pain control. In M. Weisenberg, & B. Tursky (Eds.), *Pain: New perspectives in therapy and research* (pp. 67–73). New York: Plenum Publishing Company.

Tinnermann, A., Geuter, S., Sprenger, C., Finsterbusch, J., & Buchel, C. (2017). Interactions between brain and spinal cord mediate value effects in nocebo analgesia. *Science, 358,* 105–108.

Tyler, A., & Wampold, B. E. (2012). The 2011 Leona Tyler award address: The relationship–and its relationship to the common and specific factors of psychotherapy. *The Counseling Psychologist, 40,* 601–623.

Wampold, B. E. (2015). How important are the common factors in psychotherapy? An update. *World Psychiatry, 14,* 270–277.

Watzlawick, P., Weakland, J., & Fisch, R. (1974). Change. *Principles of problem formation and problem resolution.* New York: W. W. Norton & Company.

White, M., & Epston, D. (1990). *Narrative means to therapeutic ends.* New York: W. W. Norton & Co.

White, M. (2007). *Maps of narrative practice.* New York: W. W. Norton & Co.

Yalom, I. D. (2008, 2009). *Staring at the sun. Overcoming the terror of death.* San Francisco: Jossey-Bass (A Wiley Imprint).

Yalom, I. D. (2017). *Becoming myself. A psychiatrist's memoir.* New York: Basic Books.

Zeig, J. K. (2017). *The anatomy of experiential impact through Ericksonian psychotherapy. Seeing, doing, being.* Phoenix, AZ: The Milton H. Erickson Foundation Press.

Index

Printed in the United States
By Bookmasters

Printed in the United States
By Bookmasters